D1586593

Nutrition and
Prevention and Treatment

Salah Gariballa MD, FRCP

*Clinical Senior Lecturer, The University of Sheffield and Barnsley Hospital,
Sheffield Institute for Studies on Ageing, UK*

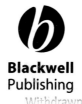

Blackwell
Publishing

Editorial Offices:
Blackwell Publishing Ltd, 9600 Garsington Road, Oxford OX4 2DQ, UK
  Tel: +44 (0)1865 776868
Blackwell Publishing Professional, 2121 State Avenue, Ames, Iowa 50014-8300, USA
  Tel: +1 515 292 0140
Blackwell Publishing Asia Pty Ltd, 550 Swanston Street, Carlton, Victoria 3053, Australia
  Tel: +61 (0)3 8359 1011

First published 2004 by Blackwell Publishing Ltd

Library of Congress Cataloging-in-Publication Data
Gariballa, Salah.
   Nutrition and stroke : prevention and treatment/Salah Gariballa.
      p. cm.
   Includes bibliographical references and index.
   ISBN 1-4051-1120-8 (alk. paper)
   1. Cerebrovascular disease–Nutritional aspects.   2. Cerebrovascular disease–Diet therapy.
   3. Cerebrovascular disease–Prevention.   I. Title.

   RC388.5.G37 2004
   616.8'10654–dc22
   2003069155

ISBN 1-4051-1120-8

A catalogue record for this title is available from the British Library

Set in 10/13pt Palatino
by DP Photosetting, Aylesbury, Bucks
Printed and bound in India
by Replika Press Pvt Ltd.

The publisher's policy is to use permanent paper from mills that operate a sustainable forestry policy, and which has been manufactured from pulp processed using acid-free and elementary chlorine-free practices. Furthermore, the publisher ensures that the text paper and cover board used have met acceptable environmental accreditation standards.

For further information on Blackwell Publishing, visit our website:
www.blackwellpublishing.com

This work is dedicated to my parents, my wife Nesrin and my children
Mohammed, Samar and Muaz

Contents

Preface

Nutrition as a science was founded by Antoine Lavoisier towards the end of the eighteenth century, but dietetics is a much older subject. Hippocrates frequently gave his patients advice about what foods they should eat, and since the days of ancient Greece, doctors in all countries have used dietetics as an important part of their treatment. From a nutritional point of view mankind can be divided into four types: (1) primitive hunter–gatherers, (2) peasants, agriculturists and pastoralists, (3) urban slum dwellers and (4) the affluent.

There are not many primitive hunter–gatherers in the world today, but societies depending on these methods were fairly common until the early part of the twentieth century. The few hunter–gatherers left nowadays live largely on vegetables and fruit with little animal food. An example is the Kung Bushmen who live in an isolated area of northern Botswana. Truswell (Truswell & Ward 1979) studied their nutrition and reported that they were rarely obese and, at the end of the dry season, tended to become undernourished. Except after illness or injury they did not experience malnutrition.

Agriculturists and pastoralists are people who stay in one place, build homes and store treasure. Great civilisations like the Egyptian, the Mayan and the classical Greeks were based on agriculture. Nutrition in this setting has fundamental differences from that of the hunter–gatherers. Peasant agriculturists were liable to develop specific deficiency diseases when a large proportion of their dietary energy came from a single staple food, such as a cereal or starchy food.

New urban dwellers were uprooted from their rural origins and packed round the factories in bad housing. Barbara Ward in 1969 described this new migrant population, crowded into towns of Africa, Asia and Latin America. Millions pile on top of one another, and the farms cannot feed them or the industries employ them. They have the worst of both worlds – old rural traditions are lost but they do not benefit from being in an urban setting.

In affluent societies such as Britain today, the malnourished segment of the community is no longer babies, who in fact tend to be obese, but some of the elderly, especially those who are failing physically or mentally. Affluence creates its own nutritional problems, and nutrition has some part to play in the genesis of diseases such as hypertension, coronary heart disease, stroke, diabetes mellitus, gallstones and cancer. Florence Nightingale wrote in her *Notes on Nursing*, published in 1859: 'Remember that sick cookery should half do the work of your patient's weak digestion. But if you further impair it with your bad articles, I know not what is to become of him or it. If the nurse is an intelligent being, and not a mere carrier of diets to and from the patient, let her exercise her intelligence in these things.'

Hippocrates documented stroke in his first account of the syndrome, using the original ancient Greek word 'apoplexia'. This implied 'being struck down violently, perhaps by lightning or a thunderbolt', and, as the Swiss doctor Wepfer discovered in 1658, mainly occurred in elderly people. Perhaps it also occurred in some, like Florence Nightingale's patients, with the sickest cookery and weakest digestion.

Salah Gariballa

Truswell, X. & Ward, X. (1979) Historical perspective. In *Human Nutrition and Dietetics*, pp. 1–5. Churchill Livingstone, Edinburgh.

Acknowledgements

I wish to express my deepest gratitude to all those who helped me with planning and carrying out the studies I have quoted in this book. Special thanks are given to the subjects who participated in these studies.

I would like to thank all the copyright holders who have kindly granted permission for their material to be used in this volume. Acknowledgements for figures and tables have been noted within the text. I would like to acknowledge here those publishers who have kindly allowed me to adapt sections of text from their publications:

Data in Chapters 2 and 3 has been adapted from Gariballa, S.E. & Sinclair, A.J. (1998). Nutrition, ageing and ill health. *British Journal of Nutrition* **80** (1), 7–23. With permission from The Nutrition Society.

Data in Chapter 4 has been reproduced from Gariballa, S.E. & Sinclair, A.J. (1997) Diagnosing undernutrition in elderly people. *Reviews in Clinical Gerontology* **7**, 367–71. With permission from Cambridge University Press.

Data in Chapter 5 is adapted from Gariballa, S.E. (2000). Nutritional factors in stroke. *British Journal of Nutrition* **84**, 5–17. With permission from The Nutrition Society.

Data in Chapter 8 is based on material from Brown, A.A. & Hu, F.B. (2001). Dietary modulation of endothelial function: implications for cardiovascular disease. *American Journal of Clinical Nutrition* **73** (4), 673–86. © American Journal of Clinical Nutrition, American Society for Clinical Nutrition.

The section on cerebral ischaemia in Chapter 9 is adapted from Gariballa, S.E. & Sinclair, A.J. (1999) Oxidative stress and cerebrovascular disease. *Reviews in Clinical Gerontology* **9**, 197–206. With permission from Cambridge University Press.

Abbreviations

AMC	Arm muscle circumference
ANOVA	Analysis of variance
BMI	Body mass index
BMR	Basal metabolic rate
BSF	Biceps skin-fold thickness
CHD	Coronary heart disease
CHI	Creatinine–height index
COMA	Committee on Medical Aspects of Food Policy
CRPs	C-reactive proteins
CSF	Cerebrospinal fluid
CVD	Cardiovascular disease
DoH	Department of Health
DXA	Dual-energy X-ray absorptiometry
EAR	Estimated average daily requirement
FAO	Food and Agriculture Organization
Fe	Iron
HDL	High density lipoprotein
HPLC	High performance liquid chromatography
ICAM-1	Intercellular adhesion molecule-1
IHD	Ischaemic heart disease
K	Potassium
LBM	Lean body mass
LDL	Low density lipoprotein
MAC	Mid-arm circumference
Mg	Magnesium
MNA	Mini nutritional assessment
NHANES	National Health and Nutrition Examination Survey
NHS	National Health Service
NMDA	N-methyl D-aspartate
NSAID	Non-steroidal anti-inflammatory drug
PACI	Partial anterior circulation infarct
PEG-tube	Percutaneous gastrostomy tube
PEU	Protein-energy undernutrition
Q1–Q3	Inter-quartile range
RDA	Recommended dietary allowance

SCALES	(S = Sadness; C = Cholesterol; A = Albumin; L = Loss of body weight; E = Eat; S = Shopping)
SD	Standard deviation
SENECA	Survey in Europe on Nutrition and the Elderly
TBARS	Thiobarbituric acid reactive substances
TBW	Total body water
TLC	Total lymphocyte count
TSF	Triceps skin-fold thickness
VCAM-1	Vascular cell adhesion molecule-1
VWF	Von Willebrand factor
WHO	World Health Organization
Zn	Zinc

I Nutrition and Ageing

1 The Challenge of Stroke

1.1 Definition

A stroke is defined as rapidly developing clinical signs of focal and, at times, global loss of cerebral function with symptoms lasting more than 24 hours or leading to death and with no apparent cause other than that of vascular origin (World Health Organization 1971).

1.2 Epidemiology

The incidence of stroke is strongly age-related, with a hundred-fold increase in incidence rates, from about 3 per 10 000 people in the third and fourth decades to almost 300 per 10 000 in the eighth and ninth decades (Bonita 1992). In other words, more than 75% of strokes occur in people aged above 65 years. The majority of strokes (about 80%) are due to cerebral infarction, 10% are due to primary intracerebral haemorrhage, 5% due to subarachnoid haemorrhage, and in 5% the cause is uncertain (Warlow et al. 1996).

1.3 The burden of stroke

Stroke is a common and devastating event, which often results in death or major loss of independence, with immense human and financial costs. Approximately 125 000 and 500 000 new or recurrent strokes occur each year in the UK and USA, respectively, accounting for around one in ten of all deaths. However, the majority of strokes are not fatal, and the major burden is long-term disability. Stroke is the third most common cause of death in most Western populations after ischaemic heart disease (IHD) and cancer (Warlow et al. 1996). It is thus the commonest life-threatening neurological disorder, and the resulting disability is the most important single cause of severe disability among Western people living in their own homes (Martin et al. 1988). It is also the second most common cause of dementia, the most common cause of epilepsy in the elderly, and a frequent cause of depression. Stroke in the developing world is less well documented; however, reports from the Asia–Pacific Consensus Forum on Stroke Management predict that 'In the next 30

3

years the burden of stroke will grow most in developing countries rather than in the developed world' (Poungvarin 1998). Treatment of stroke is expensive and may account for around 13% of the district bed-stay cost in Great Britain (Forbes 1993). Hospital care in the acute phase after stroke is the most costly component of stroke patients' care (around 7.6% of total hospital service expenditure), with the excessive length of hospital stay for a small proportion of patients explaining the high and disproportionate use of resources (Forbes 1993).

1.4   Risk factors for stroke

Several general risk factors contribute to the development and progression of atherosclerosis, and they may lead to the development of an acute stroke in a susceptible individual. These factors include hypertension, cigarette smoking, diabetes mellitus and excessive alcohol consumption, and possibly hyper-cholesterolaemia. However, there are other risk factors which are directly associated with ischaemic stroke including the presence of cerebrovascular disease, ischaemic heart disease, peripheral vascular disease, carotid artery stenosis and conditions that promote formation of cardiac emboli such as atrial fibrillation, prosthetic valves and cardiomegaly (Bamford et al. 1988).

1.5   Nutrition and risk of stroke

Modification of known risk factors such as hypertension, high cholesterol levels and smoking have been shown to be effective strategies for preventing cardiovascular diseases. However, these 'classical' risk factors, along with known non-modifiable risk factors such as age, sex and family history, cannot fully explain why some people develop myocardial infarction and stroke, while others do not (Lonn & Yusuf 1999). Additional factors may have a role in the pathogenesis of atherosclerosis. For example, recent epidemiological studies have shown that increased intake of antioxidants through diet or supplement, particularly vitamins E and C and β-carotene, is associated with a lower risk of coronary heart disease (CHD) and stroke. There is also strong epidemiological evidence that a raised homocysteine concentration, which may be related to poor dietary intake of folate, vitamins B6 and B12, is asso-ciated with increased cardiovascular risk (Lonn & Yusuf 1999). Diet may also influence stroke by affecting blood pressure or the development of athero-sclerosis. Changes in dietary habits may explain the recent fall in incidence and mortality of stroke, since eating more fresh fruit and vegetables has been found to be associated with decreased incidence of atherosclerotic diseases and prolonged lifespan (Acheson & Williams 1983). There are now important epidemiological links in stroke patients between mortality and dietary intake of sodium, potassium, calcium, magnesium and animal protein (Xie et al. 1992).

1.6 Post-stroke nutrition

Evidence exists that dietary problems not only influence the incidence of stroke but its course and outcome after the stroke has occurred. From the limited amount of research which has so far been carried out, it has been shown that a significant number of stroke patients are undernourished, not just on admission but also whilst in hospital, and their nutrition deteriorated further, especially that of those most dependent. There is a relationship between undernutrition, impaired cell-mediated response and clinically manifest infection (Chandra 1983). Undernourished stroke patients are likely to suffer more infections which is likely to lead to more dependency, prolonged hospital stay and increased cost of stroke care. There is some evidence, although incomplete, that nutritional support may reduce the length of hospital stay, morbidity and mortality in stroke patients (Nyswonger & Helmchen 1992; Gariballa et al. 1998a). Although stroke patients are particularly at risk of worsening nutritional status, the full extent of this problem and its contribution to stroke outcome is presently unknown.

Because the majority of the cost of care for elderly stroke patients is incurred in meeting in-patient and acute rehabilitation needs, nutritional manipulation during this period in particular may bring about improvement in the outcome of stroke patients and also reduce the overall cost of care. In the UK, the King's Fund report stated that the NHS could potentially save £266 million per year by improving recovery rates and shortening hospital stays through nutritional support for those patients who are known to be undernourished (Lennard-Jones 1992). A recent report has estimated that the extra cost of treating patients suffering from chronic diseases such as stroke and malnutrition, compared with those without malnutrition, may be around £7.3 million per year per 100 000 of such patients (Martyn et al. 1998).

2 Ageing Changes Relevant to Nutrition in Elderly People

2.1 Introduction

Since the early 1930s many Western societies have experienced a considerable increase in the number of elderly people. This has created a need for additional knowledge of age-related changes with respect to nutrition, which is important for the treatment and prevention of disease and for maintaining good health and quality of life in an ageing population. Ageing, disease, lifestyle and environmental factors account for many of the changes observed in older people. It is well recognised that with advancing age the incidence of chronic diseases increases substantially, and evidence points to the importance of nutrition in the development, susceptibility and outcome of these diseases. There are, however, problems in diagnosing undernutrition in the elderly because of physical and biochemical changes which may take place as part of normal ageing. Additionally, the neglect of nutritional assessment in the setting of acute clinical medicine is well known (Garrow 1994). McWhirter and Pennington (1994) reported that in Great Britain undernutrition is prevalent and largely unrecognised in hospital in-patients on admission and it tends to get worse during their hospital stay. There is no doubt that good nutrition contributes to the health and well-being of elderly people and to their ability to recover from illness (Department of Health and Social Security 1992).

2.2 Gastrointestinal tract

Ageing may be accompanied by changes in the body which may impair a person's ability to choose and prepare food and consume adequate amounts of nutrients, but such changes are complex and difficult to document. However, objective changes in smell and taste have been observed which may directly decrease food intake or alter the type of foods which are selected. With ageing there may be a progressive loss in the number of taste buds per papilla on the tongue. The taste buds remaining, which detect primarily bitter or sour tastes, show a relative increase with ageing (Schiffman 1973). In addition, the ability to identify foods while blindfolded decreases with advancing age. This is a common perceived problem among elderly individuals who complain of loss of both taste and smell (Exton-Smith 1980a). Impaired appetite is often associated with reduction in taste and smell, and this occurs in up to 50% of elderly people (Schiffman 1978; Busse 1980). Taste thresholds are higher among institutionalised than in healthy elderly men, and the use of drugs, particularly antihypertensive medication, appears to be a contributing factor (Spitzer 1988). Despite this, none of the above factors have been shown in prospective controlled studies to affect oral intake of food or nutritional status of the elderly.

Dental health is important in old age, and 74% of the elderly in England and Wales in 1978 were edentulous (Todd & Walker 1980). There is evidence linking nutritional status to dentition (McGandy et al. 1966; Department of Health and Social Security 1979a; Geissler & Bates 1984), but a causal relationship is yet to be established in randomised controlled intervention trials.

There are some documented gastrointestinal changes in the elderly that could affect their food intake. For example, changes in peristaltic activity of the oesophagus may result in delay of oesophageal emptying (Bhanthumnavin & Schuster 1977). Absorption of some nutrients, in particular vitamin B12, may be impaired because of mild ageing-related achlorhydria, but the evidence here is incomplete (Russell 1986). Southgate and Durnin (1970) found no evidence of impaired absorption between young and elderly people when they analysed the nutrient composition of food eaten and urine and faeces excreted. Some researchers have reported widespread nutritional deficiencies associated with bacterial contamination of the small bowel (Roberts et al. 1977; McEvoy et al. 1983; Haboubi & Montgomery 1992). McEvoy et al. (1983) found that 17 of 24 malnourished patients had bacterial contamination of the small bowel; Haboubi & Montgomery (1992) and Roberts et al. (1977) reported a significant improvement in nutritional status in elderly patients after treatment of bacterial contamination with antibiotics: all these elderly patients had an anatomically normal small bowel. However, these studies included non-randomly selected malnourished patients and the numbers studied were small. Lipski et al. (1992) randomly selected and studied three groups of 54 fit young subjects, 103 fit community elderly, and 73 elderly long-stay hospital patients. All subjects had simultaneous lactulose hydrogen and ^{14}C-glycocholic acid breath tests for assessment of bacterial contamination of the small bowel. Nutritional state was assessed by anthropometry (body weight, height, triceps skinfold thickness and mid-arm circumference), haematology (haemoglobin, serum B12 and red cell folate), and biochemistry (serum albumin, calcium and alkaline phosphatase). They found significantly more positive breath tests in the elderly group compared with young fit subjects, but there was no association between positive breath tests and anthropometry, haematology and biochemistry. The most likely interpretation of these apparently conflicting reports is that bacterial contamination of an anatomically normal small bowel in the elderly is the result of rather than the cause of malnutrition.

Of the studies reviewed in this latter section few have attempted to give a specific and objective definition of malnutrition. For example, in the study by Haboubi and Montgomery (1992) malnutrition was implied on the basis of hypoalbuminaemia and a skinfold thickness below the 25th percentile, although the authors did not quote the source of normative data.

The mechanisms through which malnutrition might cause bacterial growth are not fully understood, but there is evidence that the activity of several enzyme systems involved in bactericidal processes may be reduced in malnutrition (Chandra 1983).

2.3 Body mass and composition

Changes in body composition seen with ageing include a decrease in lean body mass and an increase in body fat (Forbes & Reina 1970). Decreased physical activity accounts for the increased body fat, and this may lead to decreased energy or calorie intake (Morley 1986). These changes in body composition, including those in fat distribution, may be associated with changes in various physiological functions that affect metabolism, nutrient intake, physical activity and risk of chronic disease (Chumlea et al. 1992). During ageing bone density alters, caused by decreased mineral content (Durnin & Womersley 1974). Severe osteoporosis may cause the bones in the legs to bow under the weight of the body. This bowing, combined with changes of the spine, makes measurement of height unreliable in some elderly subjects, even in those who are able to stand unaided (Miall et al. 1967). Body weight is rapidly affected by short-term changes in a person's life, in addition to the effects of acute and chronic diseases or undernutrition. Studies of body weight should be longitudinal and also take into account changes in anthropometric indices and alterations in the relative amount and anatomical distribution of adipose and muscle tissues with old age (Baumgartner 1995).

2.3.1 Assessment of body composition in elderly people

Many body composition assessment methods have limited application for the elderly. For example, underwater weighing may be unsuitable for disabled individuals, isotope dilution techniques are not universally accessible, and other models face similar limitations because they require combinations of these measurements. Many studies have been undertaken using a variety of simple bedside measurement techniques from which body composition can be predicted, but these techniques have not been validated specifically for use in elderly people. Fuller et al. (1996) have evaluated a range of body composition prediction techniques and equations against total body water (TBW), which is measured using an isotope dilution method considered to be suitable for elderly people. Body composition predictors, including body weight, height, skin-fold thickness, bioelectrical impedance and near-infrared interactance, were evaluated against TBW in 23 randomly selected men over 75 years old, and dual-energy X-ray absorptiometry (DXA) in 15 volunteers from this group. Comparisons were made between anthropometric and impedance methods for estimating limb muscle mass. They found that some body composition predictions are unacceptable (at least for TBW) in older men, and care is recommended when selecting from these methods. The authors also reported that DXA is not the most appropriate reference method for assessing muscle mass; further studies using scanning techniques, such as magnetic resonance imaging and computer-aided tomography scans, are recommended instead.

2.4 Physical activity

Reduced physical activity will obviously reduce the total energy expenditure of an individual, and this is an important factor contributing to reduced energy requirement in the elderly (Durnin & Lean 1992). However, the energy cost of normal activities has been reported to increase with age for men (Durnin 1985). In Nottingham, healthy women aged 70 years had a 20% higher energy cost for walking at a standard speed than either men of the same age or younger women (Bassey & Terry 1986, 1988). In a questionnaire survey based on a sample of the general population resident in private (non-institutional) households in Great Britain, information was collected from 3691 people aged 65 or over about participation in physical activities in the previous four weeks. In the 60–69 years age group about 70% recorded no outdoor activity and this proportion was even higher in the over 70s age group (Office of Population, Censuses and Surveys 1989).

A survey in Nottingham of the customary activity of elderly people found that the average reported daily time spent undertaking active pursuits was less than one hour, and was lower still in those aged 75 years or more (Dallosso et al. 1988); four years later a significant decline in activity levels was found in the 620 survivors (Bassey & Harries 1993).

Another feature of ageing which may restrict physical activity is the presence of a variety of degenerative and chronic diseases of which chronic obstructive airway disease, angina and arthritis are examples.

Physical activity contributes to good physical and psychological health at all ages (Royal College of Physicians 1991), and inactivity in the elderly associated with a minor illness often leads to loss of muscle tone and mass, and thereafter former physical activity levels may never be regained.

2.5 Social and medical conditions related to ageing

Decreased visual acuity, joint problems, hand tremors and hearing problems, or a combination of them, may make the task of food preparation and eating more difficult for the elderly. Other risk factors which may affect nutritional status in the elderly include isolation with an inability to go out shopping, loss of a spouse, depression and bereavement, decreased mobility, dementia, anorexia due to disease (especially cancer), medications, poor dentition or alcoholism, and most important of all acute illness (Department of Health and Social Security 1972, 1979a, b).

In institutions, lack of supervision or assistance at mealtimes may be an important factor resulting in poor food intake (Hoffman 1993). Because old people are disproportionately isolated, on low incomes or disabled, socio-economic factors and disease are likely to have more influence on their nutritional status than age alone. A report from the USA showed an increase in disability with age, from 3.5% of people aged 65–69 years who had difficulty preparing food, rising to 26.1% of those aged over 85. The percentage of people who suffered difficulty with shopping rose from 1.9% in the younger group to 37% in the older group (Dawson et al. 1987). The Nottingham Longitudinal Survey of Activity and Ageing which studied a sample of 1042 old people was thought to be representative of the elderly population in the UK in terms of social class, age, sex and the number living alone. Subjects were asked whether they did cooking and shopping: 6% of women aged 65–74 years said they did not do their own cooking, rising to 12% of women aged over 74 years; 11% of women aged 65–74 years did not do their shopping, rising to 30% for those over 74 years (Dallosso et al. 1988). Food-associated problems and perceived health may also have a role to play.

Ultimately identification of those ambulatory elderly people at risk of undernutrition requires an understanding of their social, cultural and economic environment.

2.6 Summary

Many Western societies have experienced a considerable increase in the number of elderly people. Ageing, disease, lifestyle and environmental factors account for many of the changes observed in older people. There is a growing recognition that age-related physiological anorexia may predispose to protein-energy undernutrition in the elderly, particularly in the presence of other 'pathological' factors associated with ageing, such as social, psychological, physical and medical factors, the majority of which are responsive to treatment. This has created a need for additional knowledge of age-related changes relevant to nutrition, which have importance in the treatment and prevention of diseases such as stroke and in maintaining good health and quality of life in an ageing population.

3 Macro- and Micronutrients in Elderly People

Macronutrients

3.1 Energy requirement

The scientific evidence about energy requirement in the elderly is often incomplete and highly variable. The reasons for this include paucity and variability of data on energy intake and requirements, and most important of all, diversity of physical activity patterns in the elderly population. In a series of studies, elderly subjects from the USA (McGandy et al. 1966; Uauy et al. 1978) consumed on average more energy than subjects in European studies (Durnin, 1961; Bunker & Clayton 1989; Loenen et al. 1990); however, the USA trials included fewer people than the European studies. The UK's Department of Health and Social Security longitudinal study, which examined energy intake in 365 elderly people in 1967–1968 and again five years later, found that the average energy intake had fallen from 2235 to 2151 kcal per day for men and from 1711 to 1636 kcal per day for women (Department of Health and Social Security 1979a). A similar trend for energy intakes to fall with age over five years was observed in a study of 269 elderly people in Gothenberg, Sweden (Lundgren et al. 1987).

3.2 Energy expenditure

3.2.1 Basal metabolic rate

Basal metabolic rate (BMR) reflects the energy requirements for maintenance of the intracellular environment and the mechanical processes such as respiration and cardiac function that sustain the body at rest (Heber & Bray 1980). It usually accounts for between 60 and 75% of total energy expenditure. The FAO/WHO/UNU Expert Consultation (World Health Organization 1985), used equations to predict BMR (Schofield et al. 1985). These equations may be less appropriate for elderly populations, especially those of older men, because of small numbers in the study; since then more data have been collected which have allowed a more precise estimate of current energy requirements in the elderly. BMR increases with body size, particularly with lean body mass, and this explains why it is higher in men than women, and 10–20% less in old people because of reduced muscle mass and increased fat mass with ageing (McGandy et al. 1966; Munro et al. 1987).

3.2.2 Physical activity

In most working populations, physical activity accounts for 10–35% of total energy expenditure. The energy expenditure of different activities depends on the amount of work being carried out, the body weight of the individual and the efficiency with which that work is carried out. In general, ageing is associated with a reduction in efficiency, which may make standard tasks like walking require the expenditure of up to 20% more energy in older people (Bassey & Terry 1986, 1988). This reduced efficiency may be one reason why older individuals slow down; it may contribute to negative energy balance, weight loss and undernutrition in some settings.

3.2.3 Thermogenesis

The term thermogenesis encompasses a wide variety of phenomena that include energy expenditure and heat generation associated with feeding, body temperature maintenance, and thermogenic response to various specific stimuli such as smoking, caffeine and drugs. Thermogenesis has also been postulated to play a part in the regulation of body weight. This field of research is complex in humans, and the theory is derived mainly from animal models (Durnin & Lean 1992). In the elderly, resting circulating catecholamine concentrations are elevated (Lake et al. 1977); the responsiveness to catecholamines may decline with age, as is the case in experimental animals (Rothwell & Stock 1983). Poehlman (1993) reported that the thermic response to ingestion of a meal appears to be influenced by age, physical activity and body composition.

It is possible that the fall in the capacity for thermogenesis with age may explain the increased risk of hypothermia in the elderly. However, in most cases of hypothermia there is a precipitating physical cause such as stroke, which may or may not have a direct effect on thermogenesis.

3.3 Protein requirement

There is almost a consensus regarding the current recommendation for protein intake of free living healthy elderly; this is between 0.75 and 0.8 g/kg (World Health Organization 1985; Department of Health and Social Security 1991).

Total protein contained in lean body mass falls with age, and protein synthesis, turnover and breakdown all decrease with advancing age (Golden & Waterlow 1977; Uauy et al. 1978; Lehmann et al. 1989). Based on a series of studies and a literature review, Munro and Young (1980) stated that progressive loss of protein is a major feature of ageing throughout adult life. This appears to affect some tissues, notably muscle, more than others. There is no direct evidence to suggest that this erosion of tissue protein is due to lack of adequate amounts of protein in the average diet.

Ill health, trauma, sepsis and immobilisation may upset the equilibrium between protein synthesis and degradation (Munro & Young 1980; Reeds & James 1983; Rennie & Harrison 1984; Beaumont et al. 1989; Lehmann et al. 1989). Campbell et al. (1994) studied the dietary protein requirements of 12 elderly men and women aged 56–80 years using short-term nitrogen balance techniques and calculations recommended by the Joint FAO/WHO/UNU Expert Consultation (World Health Organization 1985); they also recalculated nitrogen-balance data from three previous protein requirement studies in elderly people. From the current and retrospective data they reported that a safe protein intake for elderly adults would be 1.0–1.25 g/kg/day.

Micronutrients

3.4   Vitamins

Because of low food intake and increased incidence of physical diseases which may interfere with intake, absorption, metabolism and utilisation, vitamin deficiency is more likely in the elderly than in the young. Intake of most vitamins is reduced in smokers, and alcoholics are more likely to suffer from folate and thiamine deficiency (Ferro-Luzzi et al. 1988). Up to 50% of elderly people in populations surveyed ingested vitamin supplements, even though there is no documented benefit from this practice when the diet is adequate (Gupta et al. 1988). Brocklehurst et al. (1968) studied 80 long-term geriatric inpatients, most of whom had stroke or dementia. Patients were randomly allocated to placebo or a multivitamin supplement that contained 3 to 12 times the recommended daily allowance of thiamine, nicotinamide, riboflavin and pyridoxine plus 200 mg of ascorbic acid. Before the trial, 78% had low vitamin C status and 76% low thiamine status; at 12 months, 91% of the intervention group had normal blood levels of these vitamins compared with 14% of controls, skin haemorrhage and capillary fragility being reduced significantly in the intervention group. In a randomised double-blind placebo-controlled trial of vitamin C supplementation on 94 elderly long-term institutionalised people, Schorah et al. (1981) found that in subjects receiving the supplement there were significant gains in body weight, levels of serum albumin and pre-albumin, and in clinical rating of purpura: these studies have not been replicated. Most other studies which examined vitamin supplementation showed no statistically significant differences between supplement and placebo administration (Drinka & Goodwin 1991).

Two large surveys of vitamin status in elderly people since 1991 have improved our knowledge of this subject: the Boston Nutritional Status Survey (Hartz et al. 1992) and the Survey in Europe on Nutrition and the Elderly (Euronut SENECA Investigators 1991). Russel and Suter (1993) reviewed the literature on vitamin requirements of elderly people, including the SENECA and Boston surveys, with reference to the US National Research Council recommended dietary allowances (RDA) (National Research Council 1989). They concluded by saying, 'For now, there are data to indicate that the 1989 RDAs are too low for the elderly population (i.e. ≥ 51 years) for riboflavin, vitamin B6, vitamin D and vitamin B12, at least for certain groups of elderly people. The present RDAs for elderly people appear to be appropriate for thiamin, vitamin C and folate, but are probably too high for vitamin A. There are not enough data to make judgement on the appropriateness of the RDAs, or safe and adequate intakes for elderly people for vitamin K, niacin, biotin and pantothenic acid.'

3.4.1   Vitamins B12 and folate

The use of serum vitamin B12 to diagnose deficiency in older people is complicated by difficulties in the interpretation of low normal results. Recently, it has been shown that haematological manifestation of deficiency and the accumulation of intermediates of B12 metabolism, namely, homocysteine and methylmalonic acid, may be detected in some patients before the serum B12 concentration falls below the usual lower limit of the reference range of 150–600 pmol/l) (Metz et al. 1996). In another study the serum concentrations of vitamin B12, folate, vitamin B6 and four metabolites were measured in 99 healthy young people, 64 healthy elderly subjects and 286 elderly hospitalised patients. The prevalence of tissue deficiency of vitamin B12, folate and vitamin B6, as demonstrated by the elevated metabolite concentrations, was found to be substantially higher than that estimated by measuring concentrations of the vitamins (Joosten et al. 1993). In a prospective, multicentre, double-blind controlled study, the effect of an intramuscular vitamin supplement containing 1 mg vitamin B12, 1.1 mg folate and 5 mg vitamin B6 on serum concentrations of methylmalonic acid, homocysteine, 2-methylcitric acid and cystathionine (metabolic evidence of vitamin deficiency) in 300 elderly people with normal serum vitamin concentrations was compared with that of placebo in 175 elderly subjects living at home and 110 in hospital. The response rate to vitamin supplements suggested that metabolic evidence of vitamin deficiency is common in elderly people with normal serum vitamin levels (Naurath et al. 1995).

Homocysteine will be discussed in Chapter 7.

3.4.2   Fruit and vegetables (antioxidants)

There are several reasons why consumption of fruit and vegetables merits special attention. Besides contributing non-starch polysaccharides, they are rich sources of vitamins and minerals such as carotene, vitamins A, E, C, and potassium. Several of these micronutrients have antioxidant properties, and they may have a role in protecting against damage by oxidative free radicals, which may be involved in the mechanism of atherosclerotic injury.

In Great Britain, for example, rates of stroke and coronary heart disease (CHD) are highest in regions where consumption of fruit and vegetables is lowest; the same ecological study suggested an inverse association between fruit and vegetable consumption and incidence of stroke (Acheson & Williams 1983).

Evidence is also accumulating to show that free radical damage may be important in other diseases such as Parkinson's disease, Alzheimer's disease, chronic inflammatory disease and cancer, and that some of these diseases (cardiovascular and cancer) may be prevented or delayed to some extent by dietary changes such as reduction in fat intake and increased consumption of fruits, grains and vegetables (Halliwell 1994). Table 3.1 shows some anti-oxidants, their possible mechanism of action and also some of the recent studies in relation to oxidative stress and elderly people.

Table 3.1   Dietary antioxidants and oxidative stress (adapted from Halliwell 1994)

Constituent	Action(s)
Known to be important Vitamin E (fat soluble)	General name for group of compounds, of which α-tocopherol is most important, that inhibit lipid peroxidation. May be important in protection against cardiovascular disease. In a 2-year randomised placebo-controlled trial, 2000 IU of vitamin E per day given to patients with moderate Alzheimer's disease delayed by 50% the combined end-point of death, admission to an institution, inability to perform the activities of daily living, or severe dementia (Sano et al. 1997). In another trial, 88 healthy people aged 65 years or older were randomised to receive vitamin E (60 IU per day, 200 IU per day or 800 IU per day) or placebo. After 4 months of follow up, those who had taken vitamin E supplements showed significant improvement in the indices of immune response mediated by T cells (Meydani et al. 1997).

Contd

Table 3.1   Contd

Constituent	Action(s)
Widely thought to be important Vitamin C (ascorbic acid)	Probably assists α-tocopherol in inhibition of lipid peroxidation by recycling the tocopherol radical. Good scavenger for many free radicals and may help to detoxify inhaled oxidising air pollutants (ozone, NO_2, free radicals in cigarette smoking) in the respiratory tract. A recent cohort study in Finnish men aged over 60 has shown that vitamin C deficiency, assessed by a low plasma ascorbate concentration, is a risk factor for CHD. However, it is not known whether supplementation with vitamin C reduces the risk (Nyyssonen et al. 1997).
Probably important, but not necessarily as antioxidants β-Carotene, other carotenoids, related plant pigments	Several previous epidemiological studies suggest that high intake of such molecules is associated with diminished risk of cancer and cardiovascular disease, especially in smokers. A randomised trial in 22 071 male doctors aged 40–84 years found that β-carotene had no effect on incidence of cancer and cardiovascular disease after 14 years of follow-up (Hennekens et al. 1996). Epidemiological evidence indicates that diets high in carotenoid-rich fruits and vegetables may be associated with a reduced risk of lung cancer (Peto et al. 1981). A randomised, double-blind, placebo-controlled primary prevention trial of daily supplementation with vitamin, E, β-carotene, or both, for 5 years in a total of 29 133 male smokers aged 50–69 years from Finland and followed up for 5–8 years found no reduction in the incidence of lung cancer. In fact, this trial raises the possibility that these supplements may actually have harmful as well as beneficial effects (Alpha-Tocopherol, Beta-Carotene Cancer Prevention Study Group 1994). In the β-Carotene and Retinol Efficacy Trial, involving a total of 18 314 smokers, former smokers and workers exposed to asbestos, subjects received 30 mg of β-carotene per day and 25 000 IU of vitamin A in a randomised, double-blind, placebo-controlled design. After an average of 4 years of supplementation, the combination of β-carotene and vitamin A had no benefit and may have had an adverse effect on the incidence of lung cancer and on the risk of death from lung cancer, CVD, and any cause in smokers and workers exposed to asbestos (Omenn et al. 1996).
Possibly important Flavonoids, other plant phenolics	Plants contain many phenolic compounds that inhibit lipid peroxidation and lipoxygenases *in vitro* (e.g. flavonoids), although (similarly to ascorbate) they can sometimes be pro-oxidant if mixed with iron ions *in vitro*. How many of these products are absorbed from the gut or become available *in vivo* to act as antioxidants is unknown.

Lower antioxidant defences and increased oxidative damage may, however, be a consequence of tissue injury rather than the cause of it. Moreover, many epidemiological studies and dietary surveys, which have led to the assumption that dietary intake of essential antioxidants, such as β-carotene, vitamins A, C and E, is inversely related to the risk of stroke and CHD, have not adequately adjusted for confounding effects such as lifestyle and other environmental risk factors.

See Chapter 6 for further detailed discussion on antioxidants and risk of stroke in elderly people.

3.5 Minerals

3.5.1 Sodium (Na) and potassium (K)

Studies in hypertensive rats have found that high potassium (K) intake protects against death from stroke even though blood pressure was not affected (Tobian et al. 1985). Khaw and Barrett-Connor (1987) reported an inverse association of K intake with stroke mortality irrespective of hypertensive status. Clinical, experimental and epidemiological evidence suggests that a high dietary intake of K is associated with lower blood pressure (Langford, 1983; MacGregor, 1983; Treasure & Ploth, 1983). A major inter-population study has shown a correlation between the average sodium (Na) intake and the slope of blood pressure with age, and a negative correlation between K intake and blood pressure levels (Intersalt Cooperative Research Group 1988). Clinical studies in which manipulations of dietary Na and K have brought about changes in blood pressure in human elderly subjects support these findings (Fotherby & Potter, 1992).

Experimentally, excess salt intake has been shown to cause hypertension, not only through simple volume expansion but also through Na-accelerated vascular smooth muscle cell proliferation, and to enhance thrombosis by the acceleration of platelet aggregation (Yamori 1987).

3.5.2 Calcium (Ca) and vitamin D

There is some speculation that age-related renal impairment decreases the renal hydroxylation of vitamin D, thereby decreasing the amount of active vitamin D available for calcium absorption (Heaney et al. 1982). Many institutionalised and free living elderly (up to 50% in some studies) have inadequate vitamin D intake, and the possible causes for this include sunlight deprivation, decreased intake of dairy products, lactose intolerance and malabsorption of fat-soluble vitamins (Hoffman 1993).

Bone mass declines with age, especially in white females: this is associated with osteoporosis and an increased fracture risk. Calcium alone without oestrogens cannot fully ameliorate post-menopausal bone loss, but Ca supplementation of 1000 mg daily with exercise does slow bone loss (Prince et al. 1991). Although Ca supplementation may be necessary for certain groups of elderly people, it may be harmful in patients with a history of Ca stones, primary hyperparathyroidism, sarcoidosis or renal hypercalciuria (Heaney et al. 1982). A randomised double-blind placebo-controlled trial of the effects of three years of dietary supplementation with calcium and vitamin D in 176 men and 213 women over 65 years of age reported that dietary supplementation significantly reduced bone loss measured in femoral neck and spine and reduced the incidence of non-vertebral fractures (Dawson-Hughes et al. 1997).

3.5.3 Magnesium (Mg)

Levels of magnesium (Mg) are controlled by the kidneys and gastrointestinal tract, and appear closely linked to Ca, K and Na metabolism. Serum levels, which are those generally measured, reflect only a small part of the total body content of Mg. The intracellular content can be low, despite normal serum levels in someone with clinical Mg deficiency. Serum Mg may be of value when there are symptoms suggestive of Mg deficiency. Urine Mg analysis, especially after Mg administration, may be of value in clinical practice provided the patient's dietary history, kidney function and urine volume are taken in to account (Reinhart 1988). In patients with chest pain admitted to hospital, the frequency of hypokalaemia was found to be greater among hypomagnesaemic patients than normomagnesaemic patients (Salem et al. 1991). Stroke patients have been reported to exhibit Mg deficits in serum and CSF. Acute Mg or K deficiency can produce cerebrovascular spasm, and the lower the extracellular concentration of either Mg or K the greater the magnitude of cerebral arterial contraction (Altura et al. 1984). Potential causes of Mg deficiency, such as low dietary intake and the use of diuretic therapy, are more likely to occur in elderly people, especially those who are ill.

3.5.4 Iron (Fe)

The elderly population may have lower iron (Fe) requirements to maintain adequate status than when they were younger; those with Fe deficiency can increase their Fe absorption to the same extent as young adults (Marx 1979). However, because of a higher prevalence in elderly people of disorders which interfere with efficient Fe absorption, such as atrophic gastritis and post-gastrectomy syndromes, a proportion of elderly people have reduced dietary availability of Fe (Russell 1988). Blood loss associated with hiatus hernia, peptic ulcer, haemorrhoids and cancer, and also with non-steroidal anti-inflammatory drug (NSAID) use, is more likely in elderly people. In a study of house-bound and hospitalised elderly patients, the dietary Fe intakes were lower than the intakes of a group of free-living elderly people. However, when expressed in relation to calorie intake, the Fe densities of the diets were similar for hospitalised and free-livings subjects (Thomas et al. 1989). This finding confirms the importance of maintaining an adequate food intake if micro-nutrient needs are to be met from a normal diet.

3.5.5 Zinc (Zn)

In the UK, healthy elderly people living at home and eating a self selected diet were in metabolic balance for Zn on a mean daily intake of 137 μmol (9 mg), with leukocyte Zn levels comparable to those of healthy young people (Department of Health and Social Security 1991). Institutionalised elderly subjects are at increased risk of Zn deficiency (Thomas et al. 1988; Senapati et al. 1989).

Zinc has been found to promote healing of damaged tissues, especially skin, but only in those who are Zn deficient (Chandra 1989). Zinc is also important in cell mediated immunity: in an open and uncontrolled study a group of Zn-deficient elderly who were anergic developed positive skin tests after Zn supplementation (Wagner et al. 1983). Zinc deficiency adversely affects cellular immunity at all ages (Wagner et al. 1983; Bogden et al. 1988); however, pharmacological doses of Zn may also impair cellular immunity (Chandra, 1989).

3.6 Trace elements

Knowledge of the exact role and dietary requirements for some of the following minerals (cobalt, copper, chromium, fluoride, iodine, manganese, molybdenum and selenium) is incomplete for three reasons: they have only recently been found to be essential; dietary deficiencies of many are unknown; and the utilisation of one may be affected by the amount of other elements present. However, for some there are recommended dietary intakes which may be adequate and safe, but their optimum intakes are unknown (Ministry of Agriculture, Fisheries and Food 1995).

3.7 Summary

The majority of the stroke victims (>75%) are elderly people. There are physical, mental, social and environmental changes which take place with ageing. For example, decreased physical activity, increase in body fat, decrease in lean body mass and consequently decreased energy intake, may be associated with physiological functions that affect metabolism, nutrient intake, physical activity and risk of disease.

4 Diagnosing protein–energy undernutrition (PEU) in elderly people

4.1 Introduction

One of the greatest challenges of medicine in old age is for physicians to understand the process of ageing and to be able to distinguish it from disease, lifestyle factors and environmental exposures, the cumulative effects of which account for many of the changes observed in older people. As a result, physicians have a duty to recognise and intervene appropriately against age-related diseases. The difficulties in detecting early signs of undernutrition are similar to those encountered in the early recognition of many diseases in old age. However, in the case of nutritional deficiency there are two further difficulties: for almost every nutrient there is a long latent period before a low intake leads to overt clinical manifestations, and early diagnosis must depend upon the findings of abnormalities of special tests, including biochemical and haematological investigations; secondly, in the elderly the true significance of abnormal results of these tests is not fully understood. Many abnormalities can be related to low intake of certain nutrients, but in old age there is considerable variation between individuals. In general, in younger persons the margin of safety is wide, but in old age homeostatic mechanisms are often impaired and this precarious physiological balance may be upset by physical illness or environmental hazards to which the elderly are particularly prone (Exton-Smith 1980a).

At present, nutritional assessment has three main goals. The first is to define the type and severity of malnutrition; the second is the identification of high-risk patients; and the third is to monitor the efficacy of nutritional support. Various anthropometric, haematological, biochemical and immunological variables have been used to assess nutritional status, but the sensitivity and specificity and the relative contribution of each individual variable to the diagnostic accuracy of undernutrition have not been clearly defined. Tables 4.1 and 4.2 show some of these measures, their role in identifying patients at risk of PEU and their limitations in relation to elderly people.

Table 4.1 Assessment of nutritional status in relation to elderly people (Gariballa & Sinclair 1998a). Reproduced with permission from *British Journal of Nutrition*.

Measures of nutritional status	Comments	Limitation in elderly people
Dietary surveys, types (1) Dietary history by interview (2) Recall interviews (previous 24 h) (3) Weighted dietary intakes (4) Chemical analysis	More useful when used with social, economic, environmental, clinical and laboratory data. Dietary history or recalls give only crude information. Weighted records are most appropriate when dietary intakes are to be related to clinical findings. Chemical analysis is most accurate, but expensive and time-consuming. Evidence suggests that unbiased retrospective estimates of diet are unobtainable.	Increased age is found to be associated with decreased recall ability in some studies. Diet stability in the elderly may improve recall.

Anthropometric measurements
(1) Skeletal size (height, demispan, armspan, body weight and BMI
(2) Skin-fold thickness (triceps [TSF], biceps, subscapular, dorsum of the hand, suprailiac or thigh skin-fold thicknesses, arm fat area and waist to hip ratio)
(3) Mid-arm circumference (MAC) and arm muscle circumference (AMC)
	Total arm length and total span are reported to change with age less than height. Measurement does not need a trained observer and the subject can remain seated. Arm span approximates to height at maturity and is another alternative to measurement of height in the elderly.
	  The measurement of skin-fold thickness using constant pressure callipers provides a cheap and non-invasive assessment of subcutaneous fat. The technique is reliable in practised hands.
		Changes in the spine as a result of ageing and inability of some of the elderly to stand make height measurements alone unsatisfactory.
		  Although standards for the elderly exist for MAC and skin-fold thickness, the major difficulty is the definition of normality and referral values, and also lack of good correlation with biochemical measures.

Biochemical measures Serum albumin, transferrin, pre-albumin, retinol binding protein, ceruloplasmin plasma fibronectin and creatinine–height index (CHI) (Viteri & Alvarado 1970)	CHI may be used as an estimate of skeletal muscle mass provided renal function is stable and there is no significant element of rhabdomyolysis present, such as in septic conditions.	Values are affected by the presence of coexisting diseases and multiple drugs. Problems in collecting accurately timed urine samples, forgetfulness, dementia or incontinence make CHI measurement difficult.
Immunological measures Lymphocytopenia and anergy to skin tests	There is some evidence to support a causal relationship between malnutrition, impaired cell-mediated response and infections.	The similarity of the effects of ageing and malnutrition on immune function places the usefulness of routine immunological testing in this population in question.
Clinical assessment scales (1) History and physical examinations (2) Mini nutritional assessment (MNA) (Guigoz et al. 1994) (3) SCALES (Morley 1993)	MNA is said to be a simple and quick screening tool. It includes: anthropometric measurements, dietary questionnaire, global and subjective assessment. SCALES (S = sadness, C = cholesterol, A = albumin, L = loss of body weight, E = eat, S = shopping) is reported to have high sensitivity to detect people potentially at risk of malnutrition.	History and examination may be as effective as other objective measurements. MNA and SCALES have not been tested on a wider scale.

Table 4.2 Nutritional assessment aims and limitations (Gariballa & Sinclair 1998a). Reproduced with permission from *British Journal of Nutrition.*

Aims	Measures used to assess nutritional status	Limitations
Definining type and severity of malnutrition	Clinical assessment (history and physical examination). The simplest way is to ask about unintentional weight loss Anthropometric: body weight, body weight to height ratio, triceps skin-fold thickness, arm muscle area and arm fat area Biochemical: serum albumin concentration is the most widely used. To a lesser extent transferrin, pre-albumin, retinol binding protein and ceruloplasmin are used (Dionigi et al. 1986).	May be as effective as other objective measurements. Needs to be studied more scientifically. Lack of definition of normality or referral data. May vary between and within populations. No single biochemical indicator has proved better than any other (Dionigi et al. 1986). Variation may be due to causes other than malnutrition, such as abnormal distribution in the extravascular space, or increased catabolism, or net loss, disease process, or a combination.
Identification of high risk patients	Different combinations of several markers have been proposed by various workers. Buzby et al. (1979) identified four related factors (serum albumin, serum transferrin, triceps skin-fold thickness and delayed hypersensitivity). Klidjian et al. (1982) have shown that reduced arm muscle circumference and impaired skeletal function measured by forearm muscle dynamometry are positively correlated with an increased risk of post-operative complications.	Standardised nutritional variables are not yet available in clinical practice. The factors determining the risk of malnutrition are many and interrelated, and include the patient's previous nutritional status, the disease process itself, and the magnitude and anticipated duration of associated catabolic stresses (Souba 1997).
Monitoring the efficacy of nutritional support	Selected biochemical variables such as serum albumin concentration, pre-albumin concentration, transferrin value, retinol binding protein value and fibronectin[a] are used to determine if a patient is responding to the nutritional support programme. Maintenance of a positive nitrogen balance and body weight gain may be useful as well.	Monitoring should be more intensive in the early phases and major functions (renal, hepatic, cardiovascular) should be evaluated. Monitoring the efficacy of nutritional support is difficult and controversial. Different centres use different approaches (Dionigi et al. 1986).

[a] Fibronectin is an opsonic glycoprotein. During starvation values fall by 25–30%. Has been proposed as a sensitive index of nutritional depletion and repletion (Howard et al. 1984).

4.2   Methods used to assess nutritional status

4.2.1   Dietary surveys

Dietary surveys cannot be used alone to assess nutritional status. They can, however, be used together with social, economic, environmental, clinical and laboratory data. Their main objective is to discover the food intake of individuals or groups of individuals, translate this into energy and nutrients, and relate it to the state of health. The degree of precision of the data will depend on the purpose of the survey and the method used.

It is generally agreed that chemical analysis gives the most accurate result, but this is time-consuming, expensive and difficult. For practical purposes, this method is usually appropriate in an institutional environment or where very small numbers are involved.

The weighted dietary record method may be the most appropriate when dietary intakes are to be related to clinical findings. If crude information is required, then a dietary history or the recall method may suffice. Friedenreich et al. (1992) reviewed 17 studies, which have all examined either the validity (three studies) or the reliability (14 studies) of retrospective dietary reporting. They concluded that the current diet exerted a strong influence on the recall of the past diet, and the correlation coefficient between original and recalled diets decreased as the time interval between the diet assessments increased. There was no difference in recall ability by sex, but increased age was found to be associated with decreased recall reliability in some studies. In another extensive review of dietary assessment techniques, Bingham (1987) reported that the coefficients of variation of differences, incurred from asking subjects to estimate the weight of food portions, rather than weighing them, were in the 50% range for foods and 20% for nutrients. Accumulating evidence suggests that unbiased retrospective estimates of diet are unobtainable (Bingham, 1987; Friedenreich et al. 1992).

Many researchers have used a combination of two or more of the dietary assessment methods, developed after extensive pilot studies and shown to be workable in the elderly (Exton-Smith 1980b; Horwath 1993). There is a consensus that a quantitative record reinforced by a dietary history may be the most appropriate method when dealing with an elderly population, but the results are likely to be influenced by the duration of the dietary survey and the cognitive function in this population.

4.2.2   Anthropometric measurements

Generally, there is loss of stature, decrease in body weight, loss of bone and muscle tissue, and there may be a change in skin texture as people grow older

(Garth & Young 1956; Forbes & Reina 1970; Knight & Eldridge 1984). These losses may be universal, but their expression, progression and prevalence varies considerably within and between groups of elderly people of similar or different genetic backgrounds.

Anthropometric measurements include body weight and body weight to height ratio, arm length, forearm length, knee height, demispan and arm span; triceps, biceps, subscapular, dorsum of the hand, suprailiac, and thigh skin-fold thickness; mid-arm circumference, arm muscle area, arm fat area and waist to hip ratio. Those most commonly used are body weight, body weight to height ratio, triceps skin-fold thickness, and mid-arm circumference, arm muscle area and arm fat area; however, for the elderly, special considerations apply and these are listed here.

1. Height

Assessment of skeletal size from height alone is probably unsatisfactory for old people because of the changes which take place in the spine as a result of ageing, and the inability of some of the elderly to stand (Miall et al. 1967).

2. Demispan

Demispan is the measurement from the web between the fingers along the outstretched arm to the sternal notch with the arm in the coronal plane. The wrist is kept in neutral rotation and flexion. Total arm length and total span are reported to change with age considerably less than height (Bassey 1986). Measurement does not need a trained observer and the subject can remain seated.

3. Arm span

Arm span approximates to height at maturity and is another alternative to measurement of height in the elderly; it is found to be a reliable and practical estimate of height in non-ambulant elderly people and could be used instead of height in the determination of body mass index (BMI) (Kwok & Whitelaw 1991).

4. Body mass index (BMI)

BMI (body weight in kg divided by height in m^2) is the most common ratio used in adults. The published norms assume that lean mass is proportional to skeletal size and only fat varies (Rolland-Cachera et al. 1991). Demispan or arm span could equally well be used to assess BMI instead of height (Bassey 1986; Kwok & Whitelaw 1991).

5.   *Skin-fold thickness*

The fat mass of the body can be estimated using a variety of direct and indirect techniques (Durnin & Lean 1992). None of these methods is ideal and none refers to any gold standard of actual body fat measurement, the most reliable of which is underwater weight and densitometry using the principle of Archimedes, provided that allowance is made for the gas volume within the airways. No currently available method is sufficiently sensitive to monitor small changes within individuals, although the recently developed dual X-ray absorptiometry techniques offer some potential.

The measurement of skin-fold thickness using constant pressure callipers at standard sites on the body provides a cheap and non-invasive assessment of subcutaneous fat. The technique is reliable in practised hands, with a coefficient of variation of about 6%. Skin-fold thickness measurements in elderly people offer only a rough guide to body fatness, and must be assessed in conjunction with other indicators (Department of Health and Social Security 1992).

6.   *Mid-arm circumference (MAC)*

MAC provides a good index of whole-body skeletal muscle mass (Shenkin & Steele 1978). The measurement is usually taken at the mid-position between the olecranon and the acromial process using a flexible or rigid plastic tape. Arm muscle circumference (AMC) and arm muscle area are calculated from MAC and triceps skin-fold thickness [AMC = MAC − (TSF × 0.314)]. Although standards for the elderly exist for MAC and skin-fold thickness, the major difficulty is the definition of normality and referral values, and also lack of good correlation with biochemical measures (Frisancho 1984).

4.2.3   Clinical laboratory tests

Many biochemical parameters have been shown to be affected by age. The alterations that occur, however, are not as easily delineated as the physical changes associated with the ageing process. Interpretation of various biochemical measurements is made difficult by the presence of coexisting diseases and multiple drugs.

A broad spectrum of biochemical variables has also been advocated to provide useful nutritional information. No single indicator has proved better than others; nevertheless, serum albumin concentration is the most widely used parameter. The synthesis of albumin is known to be depressed during undernutrition and under catabolic conditions. It is well known that undernutrition affects protein synthesis negatively, and it has been shown in man that nutrition is probably the single most important factor regulating albumin synthesis (Rothschild et al. 1972a, b). As a general index of nutritional status, Mitchell and Lipschitz (1980) found serum albumin a reliable measurement in geriatric patients as well as in all other undernourished patients.

Another protein commonly used to assess visceral protein status is serum transferrin. Transferrin has a short half-life, and nutritional depletion may result in depressed levels of transferrin before any changes in the serum albumin can occur. Care must be taken when using this measurement in the aged population, since many factors can affect serum transferrin levels; for example, iron deficiency increases transferrin levels while anaemia of chronic disease decreases them (Mitchell & Lipschitz 1982a). To a lesser extent, the concentrations of pre-albumin, retinol binding protein and ceruloplasmin have also been used in nutritional assessment.

Plasma fibronectin has recently been included in the nutritional assessment of undernourished patients. It is an opsonic glycoprotein of relative molecular mass 440 000. Fibronectin depletion correlates with reticuloendothelial (RE) phagocytic clearance depression, and restoration of circulatory concentrations is associated with restoration of RE function. Opsonic fibronectin deficiency exists in septic injured patients with host defence failure. It has been shown that during starvation serum fibronectin values fall by 20–30% and after re-feeding increase to normal. For this reason, fibronectin has also been proposed as a sensitive index of nutritional depletion and repletion (Dionigi et al. 1986).

Measurements of urinary creatinine excretion may be used to estimate skeletal muscle mass, provided renal function is stable and there is no significant element of rhabdomyolysis present, such as in septic conditions. The use of the creatinine–height index (CHI) as a nutritional assessment tool has, however, been criticised because of problems involved in collecting accurately timed urine samples, forgetfulness, dementia, incontinence or contamination with faeces in the elderly (Viteri and Alvarado, 1970; Mitchell & Lipschitz 1982b).

Lymphocytopenia and anergy to skin tests have commonly been used as indicators of PEU. However, every immunological abnormality described in undernutrition has also been documented in the elderly and ascribed to the effects of senescence (Mitchell & Lipschitz 1982b). The similarity of the effects of the ageing process and of PEU on immune function places the usefulness of routine immunological testing in this population in question (Mitchell & Lipschitz 1982b), but there is evidence to support a causal relationship between undernutrition, impaired cell mediated response and infections (Chandra 1983).

Haemoglobin and haematocrit are often used to assess nutritional status, because anaemia is frequently associated with undernutrition. There is also some evidence that the anaemia related to PEU is of a unique type. Since anaemia of undernutrition is frequently due to iron or folate deficiency, assessment of these two items is important (Mitchell & Lipschitz 1982a).

4.2.4   General assessment

Nutritional assessment should always include information about social and environmental factors, and physical and mental disorders affecting the individual. Adverse social and environmental factors include ignorance, poverty and unfavourable social circumstances, especially those associated with social isolation and loneliness, lack of help and inadequate cooking facilities (Exton-Smith 1980a). Drug history and physical examination can provide valuable information about the general health and nutritional status of an individual.

Guigoz et al. (1994) have developed and validated a new nutritional assessment and screening tool known as the mini nutritional assessment (MNA); they report that it is simple and quick to perform, taking less than 10 minutes. It includes anthropometric measurements, a dietary questionnaire, and global and subjective assessment (self-perception of health and nutrition). Another nutritional screening test for physicians and dieticians is SCALES (S = sadness, C = cholesterol, A = albumin, L = loss of body weight, E = eat; S = shopping), which is said to have a high sensitivity to detect people potentially at risk of undernutrition (Morely 1993).

One way of assessing the value of these tests as useful screening tools in the detection of early undernutrition is for them to be integrated into geriatric assessment programmes. This can only be achieved if physicians are made aware that undernutrition adversely affects the prognosis of patients in the community, the acute hospital, and in geriatric evaluation and assessment units (Morley 1994).

It is well recognised that with advancing age there is a high incidence of chronic diseases, and evidence points to the importance of nutrition in the occurrence, susceptibility and outcome of these diseases. All of the clinically available nutrition screening instruments lack sensitivity and specificity, and cannot be relied on individually as definitive diagnostic tests for protein–energy malnutrition. However, in combination they are accepted measurements of nutritional status.

4.3   PEU, ill-health and outcome

The identification of PEU has serious implications during ill-health, even though abnormal nutritional indicators may reflect effects of age, functional disability, or severe underlying disease. Therefore, it remains to be determined to what extent non-nutritional factors, such as the number and severity of comorbid conditions, are the cause of both apparent poor nutrition and poor clinical outcome. As well as the possible effects of illness on nutritional status, many drugs commonly used in the elderly may have specific effects on nutrition (Durnin & Lean 1992); a list of the more common interactions is shown in Table 4.3.

Table 4.3 Some drugs which may interfere with nutritional status in elderly people (Durnin & Lean 1992).

	Increase	Decrease
Energy intake (appetite/absorption)	Phenothiazines Tricyclic antidepressants Corticosteroids	Metformin Digoxin Many antibiotics Anticancer drugs Most analgesics Theophylline
Vitamins		Isoniazid (Pyridoxine) Metformin (folate, B12) Phenothiazines (folate) Tricyclics (folate) Methotrexate (folate) Colchicine (B12) Cholestyramine (A, B12, D, E, K) Tetracycline (C) Aspirin (C) Corticosteroids (C) Anticoagulants (D, folate)
Minerals and electrolytes	Amiloride (K) Spironolactone (K) Corticosteroids (Na) Phenylbutazone (Na) Carbenoxolone (Na) Ethanol (Fe)	Diuretics (Na, K, Ca, Mg, Zn) Phosphates (Fe) Tetracycline (Fe) Antacids (Fe) NSAIDs (Fe) Iron supplements (Zn)

Key: Vitamins A, C, D, E, K, B12; sodium (Na), potassium (K), calcium (Ca), magnesium (Mg), iron (Fe), zinc (Zn) and non-steroidal anti-inflammatory drugs (NSAIDs).

In 1988, Dempsey et al. carried out a chronological review of studies relating poor nutritional status to increased surgical morbidity. Their review included retrospective and/or non-randomised trials. They found that although many studies did not control for non-nutritional variables and some were poorly defined, the evidence is overwhelmingly in favour of a strong association between poor nutritional status and poor outcome in surgical patients. In a recent study of the relationship between nutritional status and hospital outcome, Sullivan and Walls (1994) randomly selected and studied 350 admissions to a geriatric rehabilitation unit and reported that PEU (discharge serum albumin less than 35 g/l, and body weight less than 90% of ideal) appears to be a strong independent risk factor for in-hospital mortality. Several other studies of acute care hospital and institutionalised patients have demonstrated a strong correlation between PEU and an increased risk for subsequent in-hospital morbid events (Keller 1995; Muhlethaler et al. 1995; Potter et al. 1995).

4.4   Specific markers of PEU and outcome

4.4.1   Body weight

There is evidence of an association between the levels of specific clinical markers of PEU and increased risks of morbidity and mortality. For example, there have been several studies which showed strong association between body weight and mortality (Tayback et al. 1990; Manson et al. 1995; Muhlethaler et al. 1995; Potter et al. 1995). In a prospective study of undernourished elderly people in a chronic care hospital in Canada in 1995, Keller reported that an increase of at least 5% of body weight is associated with a decreased incidence of death and may reduce morbidity. Tayback et al. (1990) analysed BMI data for 4710 white, US National Health and Nutritional Examination Survey respondents aged 55 to 75 years for the period 1971 to 1975, in relation to their survival over an average of 8.7 years of follow-up; after controlling for elevated blood pressure, smoking and poverty, they found low body weight to be associated with increased mortality.

4.4.2   Serum albumin

Measurement of the serum albumin concentration has been found to be one of the best single predictors of morbidity and mortality among the aged (Mitchell & Lipschitz 1982a, b; Agarwal et al. 1988). A study (Sahyoun et al. 1996) in which 287 community-dwelling and 176 institutionalised people aged 60 years and over were followed up for 9 to 12 years after nutritional assessment showed that after controlling for age, blood urea, triglyceride, history of disease and ability to shop, the risk of mortality for subjects with albumin values of 40 g/l and over was 0.46 of the risk for those with albumin values below 40 g/l; albumin predicted long-term mortality among non-institutionalised subjects and short-term mortality among institutionalised subjects. Reinhardt et al. (1980) studied 509 hospitalised veterans with an average age of 59 years and reported that those with serum albumin concentrations greater than 35 g/l had a mortality of 1.7%, those with levels less than 34 g/l had a 25% mortality rate, and levels less than 20 g/l resulted in 62% mortality rate. Rudman et al.

(1987) also found a relationship between mortality and decreased serum albumin concentrations in undernourished elderly male patients residing in long-term institutions. Hypoalbuminaemia ($< 35\,g/l$) has been reported to be powerful indicator of an increased risk of perioperative complications in elderly patients undergoing cardiac surgery (Rich et al. 1989). A retrospective study of 79 stroke rehabilitation patients found that low serum albumin levels on admission were significantly related to poor outcome during the hospital stay (Aptaker et al. 1994). Unfortunately, most of these studies failed to control for the effect of non-nutritional confounding variables on clinical outcome.

Albumin concentrations have long been used as a measure of health and disease (Rothschild et al. 1972a). Many factors, such as PEU, catabolism, liver and renal disease, may reduce serum albumin levels (Rothschild et al. 1972b). The catabolic state and the associated neuroendocrine response which is likely to follow the acute illness may lead to altered serum albumin levels. Hypoalbuminaemia may also represent a metabolic response to severe stress, such as extensive burns or prolonged sepsis. A decrease in serum albumin after acute stress represents decreased liver biosynthesis and turnover (Rothschild et al. 1972a, b). It is therefore possible that in catabolic states the synthesis of acute phase proteins has priority over that of serum albumin, and this may partly account for some of the features of the plasma protein profile observed during the acute phase response after injury (Dionigi et al. 1986).

4.4.3   Total lymphocyte count (TLC)

A low TLC is often associated with decreased serum albumin values; yet when considered alone, TLC is a poor prognostic indicator, possibly reflecting changes in immunological function secondary to PEU. Seltzer et al. (1979) studied albumin and TLC in 500 consecutive hospital admissions and noted a 7.6% incidence of abnormal albumin and 30.2% incidence of abnormal TLC. Abnormal TLC was associated with four-fold increase in deaths, and abnormal albumin was associated with both a six-fold increase in death and complications. In combination, abnormal TLC and albumin resulted in an eight-fold increase in complication rate with a nine-fold increase in mortality, but despite mild undernutrition in patients with anergy, nutritional support has failed to correct the response and the cellular immune dysfunction (Christou et al. 1995).

There are many studies which have demonstrated a strong relationship between PEU or its markers and morbidity and/or mortality in acute and non-acute hospital settings, but a causal relationship cannot be assumed without properly designed nutrition intervention studies.

4.5 Summary

Problems in diagnosing undernutrition in the elderly are common because of physical and biochemical changes which may take place as part of normal ageing processes; in addition, overt clinical signs of undernutrition may be late to appear and much subclinical damage may have gone uncorrected. All the clinically available nutrition screening instruments lack sensitivity and specificity, and cannot be relied on individually as definitive diagnostic tests for PEU. However, in combination, these screening instruments together with clinical assessment, food frequency questionnaires, and selected anthropometric, haematological and biochemical variables, are accepted measurements of nutritional status. Of particular importance are involuntary body weight changes or values below an established population standard, arm muscle circumference, skinfold measurement and depressed secretory proteins.

II Nutritional Factors and Risk of Stroke

5 The Role of Dietary and Nutritional Factors in Stroke Prevention

5.1 Introduction

A steady fall in mortality rates from cerebrovascular disease has been observed over at least three decades in Great Britain, and for much longer in the USA. Although improvement in the rate of detection and treatment of established risk factors such as hypertension is part of the reason for the fall, no satisfactory explanation has so far been given (Vartiainen et al.1995). Data from epidemiological studies suggest that immigrants rapidly take on the stroke incidence rates of their adopted country (Syme et al. 1975). 'Classical' risk factors, such as blood pressure, cholesterol level and smoking, together with known non-modifiable risk factors such as age, sex and family history, cannot fully explain why some people develop stroke and myocardial infarction while others do not (Gordon et al. 1974; Goldman & Cook 1984; Verschuren et al. 1995). Additional factors may have a role in the pathogenesis of athero-sclerosis; for example, recent epidemiological studies have shown that increased intake of antioxidants through diet or supplement, particularly vitamins E and C and β-carotene, is associated with a lower risk of stroke and coronary heart disease (CHD). Well documented changes in eating habits, among them an increase in intake of fruit and vegetables (vitamin C) and a fall in salt intake are known to have taken place over the last four decades or longer (Acheson & Williams 1983). Thus environmental factors, including diet, may be important in the genesis of stroke and in the potential to prevent its occurrence.

5.2 Role of nutritional factors in stroke incidence and outcome

5.2.1 Fruit and vegetables (antioxidants)

Many epidemiological studies from all over the world have led to the assumption that vegetable-rich diets are associated with a higher life expectancy; antioxidants could be of principal importance in conferring the benefits of vegetable-rich diets. The role of antioxidants in the prevention and treatment of ischaemic stroke will be discussed in Chapters 6 and 9, respectively.

5.2.2 Potassium

Increased potassium intake, which results from eating more fruit and vegetables, is likely to be beneficial. Studies in hypertensive rats have found that a high potassium intake protects against death from stroke, even though blood pressure is not affected (Tobian et al. 1985). Khaw and Barrett-Connor (1987) reported an inverse association of potassium intake, irrespective of hypertensive status, with stroke mortality in a population-based cohort study in southern California. A study by Gariballa et al. (1997) found that hypokalaemia and lower 24-hour urine excretion of potassium were more common in stroke patients than control groups, and hypokalaemia post-stroke was associated with poor outcome. Clinical, experimental and epidemiological evidence suggests that a high dietary intake of potassium is associated with lower blood pressure, which is the most important known risk factor for stroke (Langford 1983; MacGregor 1983).

There is also evidence from interpopulation and clinical studies, as well as controlled clinical trials, which links diets high in sodium and low in potassium with increased blood pressure. A major interpopulation study has shown a correlation between the average sodium intake and the slope of blood pressure with age, and a negative correlation between potassium intake and blood pressure levels (Intersalt Cooperative Research Group 1988). These findings were confirmed and strengthened by further analysis of the available data from all studies worldwide (Department of Health and Social Security 1992). Clinical studies in which manipulations of dietary sodium and potassium have brought about changes in blood pressure in elderly human subjects provide further evidence that high potassium intake may protect against stroke (Fotherby & Potter 1993).

5.3 Serum albumin

High serum albumin levels within the normal range have been associated with reduced cardiovascular mortality and CHD in several reports (Phillips et al. 1989; Kuller et al. 1991; Gillum & Makuc 1992). Protein deficiency and low serum albumin concentrations have been considered as possible initiators or factors influencing atherosclerosis (Kuller et al. 1991; Gillum & Makuc 1992). Low intake of animal protein has also been suggested as a risk factor for haemorrhagic stroke in Japan (Kimura et al. 1972).

Beamer et al. (1993) conducted a prospective study in which three groups of subjects, assigned to a high or low albumin–globulin ratio of above or below 1.45, were followed up for an average of 1.5 ± 0.8 years to ascertain vascular end-points: group 1 consisted of 126 patients with acute ischaemic stroke, group 2 comprised 109 controls matched for age and clinical risk factors for stroke, and group 3 comprised 84 healthy volunteers matched for age with groups 1 and 2. Significantly increased risk for subsequent vascular events in stroke patients and in subjects with clinical risk factors for stroke was associated with a prothrombotic shift in the concentrations of blood proteins characterised by lower levels of albumin and an increased concentration of globulins and fibrinogen.

Data from the First US National Health and Nutrition Examination Survey (NHANES 1) Epidemiologic Follow-up Study (Gillum et al. 1994) were used to assess serum albumin levels as a risk factor for stroke. Over a follow-up period of 9–16 years white men aged 65–74 years with serum albumin concentrations above 44 g/l had a risk of stroke incidence only about two-thirds that of men with serum albumin concentrations below 42 g/l; this effect persisted after controlling for multiple stroke risk variables (relative risk = 0.61; 95% CI, 0.41–0.89). A similar association with stroke death was found in white men aged 65–74 years. Serum albumin was not associated with stroke risk in white women aged 65–74 years. In black people aged 45–74 years, serum albumin concentrations above 44 g/l were associated with a risk of stroke incidence only one-half and a risk of stroke death only one-quarter that seen at levels below 42 g/l after controlling for other risk variables.

The results of these studies and the association between serum albumin and stroke incidence and death need confirmation in further prospective randomised controlled studies. Nevertheless, there is sufficient evidence to suggest that low serum albumin is strongly linked with stroke incidence and outcome. The mechanism for the effect is debatable: diets low in protein and imbalanced in their protein to energy ratios can result in low serum albumin. However, inflammatory mechanisms associated with sub-clinical disease are more likely to be the initiators of the low serum albumin concentrations in the large population studies of Phillips et al. (1989), Kuller et al. (1991) and Gillum & Makuc (1992). The cause of low serum albumin, nevertheless, does not detract from its usefulness as a predictor of disease, or of situations where clinical or dietary intervention might be usefully targeted.

5.4 Hyperhomocysteinaemia

Hyperhomocysteinaemia may be common in the general population and has been linked with cardiovascular diseases. Stroke patients frequently manifest moderate hyperhomocysteinaemia; however, this may be an acute-phase response (Lindgren et al. 1995). A number of studies have shown inverse relationships of blood homocysteine concentrations with plasma/serum levels of folic acid, vitamin B6 and vitamin B12 (Kang et al. 1987; Selhub et al. 1993; Robinson et al. 1998). Folate status is an important factor in the development of hyperhomocysteinaemia, and low serum folate concentration has been found to be a risk factor for ischaemic stroke (Giles et al. 1995; Molloy et al. 1997). Further discussion on homocysteine as a risk factor for stroke is in Chapter 7.

5.5   Dietary salt, calcium, magnesium and fibre

Experimental and epidemiological studies have indicated that genetic–environmental or more particularly genetic–nutritional interaction is involved in the pathogenesis of hypertension and stroke. While hypercholesterolaemia is the major risk factor for atherosclerosis and myocardial infarction, hypertension and thrombosis are the major risks for both haemorrhagic and thrombotic stroke caused by arterionecrotic or arteriosclerotic lesions in intracerebral arteries. These pathogenic changes have been shown to be influenced by environmental and nutritional factors of which excess dietary salt is one. Experimentally, excess salt intake causes hypertension, not only through simple volume expansion but also through sodium-accelerated vascular smooth muscle cell proliferation, and enhances thrombosis by the acceleration of platelet aggregation (Yamori 1987). Moreover, Yamori et al. (1994) have shown that there are protective nutritional factors, such as potassium, calcium, magnesium, dietary fibres, protein, some amino acids and some fatty acids, which counteract the adverse effects of sodium or cholesterol intake together with other basic pathogenic processes in hypertension, atherosclerosis and thrombosis. They also stated that well balanced supplies of such beneficial dietary factors could thus be expected to aid prevention of stroke and major cardiovascular diseases.

Ascherio et al. (1998) recently studied the effects of potassium, magnesium, calcium, and fibre on stroke risk among men (n = 43 738) participating in the US Health Professionals Follow-Up Study. The age-adjusted relative risk of total stroke for men in the top quintile of potassium intake (median 4.3 g/day) compared with those in the bottom quintile (median 2.4 g/day) was 0.59 (p = 0.004); the corresponding numbers for total fibre, magnesium and calcium intake were 0.57 ($p < 0.001$), 0.62 ($p < 0.002$) and 0.78 (n.s.), respectively. This study suggests that the consumption of a diet rich in potassium, magnesium and fibre protects against stroke death in men, the protective effects being seen particularly in hypertensive subjects, but also at all blood pressures and remaining significant after adjustment for blood pressure (Ascherio et al. 1998; Suter 1999).

5.6   Dietary fat and serum lipids

There have been conflicting reports about the relationship between dietary fat intake, serum lipids and stroke incidence (Kagan et al. 1985; McGee et al. 1985). In a huge multiple risk factor intervention trial, 350 977 men aged 35–57 years, were followed up for 12 years using a single standardised measurement of serum cholesterol and other CHD risk factors; 21 499 deaths were identified. A strong positive association was evident between serum cholesterol level and death from CHD; no association was noted between serum cholesterol and stroke, but levels below 4.14 mmol/l were associated with a two-fold increase in risk of cerebral haemorrhage, increased death from cancer of the liver and pancreas, suicide and alcohol dependence (Neaton et al. 1992). A recent overview of randomised trials of cholesterol lowering and stroke incidence, which included more than 36 000 individuals, failed to show significant reduction in fatal or non-fatal stroke (Hebert et al. 1995).

In contrast, a Danish study (Lindenstrom et al. 1994) of 19 698 women and men at least 20 years old who had been randomly selected and followed up for 12 years during which non-fasting plasma lipids were measured at 5-year intervals together with cardiovascular examination, recorded 660 non-haemorrhagic and 33 haemorrhagic strokes. Total cholesterol was positively associated with risk of non-haemorrhagic stroke, but only for levels above 8 mmol/l, corresponding to the upper 5% of the distribution in the study population; plasma triglyceride concentration was significantly positively associated with risk of non-haemorrhagic events, and there was a negative, log-linear association between high-density lipoprotein cholesterol and risk of non-haemorrhagic events. Moreover, Gillman et al. (1997), in a study of 832 middle-aged US men during 20 years of follow-up (The Framingham Heart Study), found that low intakes of fat, saturated fat, and monounsaturated fat were associated with reduced risk of ischaemic stroke. A comprehensive review article on cholesterol and stroke (Evans & Fotherby 1999) stated that, although the association between cholesterol and stroke has been a contentious issue, more recent studies considering non-haemorrhagic stroke and lipid sub-fractions provide more evidence for a weak relationship between these two variables, particularly an inverse association of high density lipoprotein (HDL) cholesterol with non-haemorrhagic stroke. There are many confounding variables which may obscure any relationship between cholesterol and certain stroke sub-types.

Meta-analysis of controlled trials in patients with hyperlipidaemia has suggested that statins significantly reduce the risk of stroke, by around 30% when used in the secondary prevention of complications of atherosclerosis (Crouse et al. 1997; Herbert et al. 1997).

Further evidence of an association between stroke and cholesterol has more convincingly been demonstrated by recent intervention trials using statins. How much of the benefit of statins is independent of cholesterol lowering is unclear, but their use would seem justified in certain persons at high risk of ischaemic heart disease (IHD) and/or stroke, particularly those with existing evidence of IHD (Evans & Fotherby 1999).

5.7 Fish consumption

High levels of fish consumption have been associated with low incidence of ischaemic stroke (Gillum et al. 1996), but a similar cohort study found that ischaemic stroke rates were highest in the subgroup reporting the highest fish intake (Orencia et al. 1996). Another significant ecological study using data from 36 countries reported that fish consumption is associated with a reduced risk of death from all-causes, IHD and stroke (Zhang et al. 1999). In the prospective cohort Nurses' Health Study, Iso et al. (2001) examined the association between fish and omega-3 polyunsaturated fatty acid intake and risk of stroke sub-types: 79 839 women aged 34 to 59 years in 1980, who were free from previously diagnosed cardiovascular disease, cancer and history of diabetes and hypercholesterolaemia, and who completed a food frequency questionnaire including consumption of fish and other frequently eaten foods were followed up for 14 years. The main outcome measures were relative risk of stroke in 1980–1994 compared by category of fish intake and quintile of omega-3 polyunsaturated fatty acid intake. After 1 086 261 person-years of follow-up, 574 strokes were documented, including 119 subarachnoid haemorrhages, 62 intraparenchymal haemorrhages, 303 ischaemic strokes (264 thrombotic infarctions among which were 90 large-artery occlusive infarctions and 142 lacunar infarctions, and 39 embolic infarctions), and 90 strokes of undetermined type. Compared with women who ate fish less than once per month, those with higher intake of fish had a lower risk of total stroke: the multivariate relative risks (RRs), adjusted for age, smoking, and other cardiovascular risk factors, were 0.93 (95% confidence interval [CI], 0.65–1.34) for fish consumption one to three times per month, 0.78 (95% CI, 0.55–1.12) for once per week, 0.73 (95% CI, 0.47–1.14) for two to four times per week, and 0.48 (95% CI, 0.21–1.06) for five or more times per week (P for trend, 0.06). Among stroke sub-types, a significantly reduced risk of thrombotic infarction was found among women who ate fish twice or more per week (multivariate RR, 0.49; 95% CI, 0.26–0.93). Women in the highest quintile of intake of long-chain omega-3 polyunsaturated fatty acids had reduced risk of total stroke and thrombotic infarction, with multivariate RRs of 0.72 (95% CI, 0.53–0.99) and 0.6 (95% CI, 0.42–1.07), respectively. When stratified by aspirin use, fish and omega-3 polyunsaturated fatty acid intakes were inversely associated with risk of thrombotic infarction, primarily among women who did not regularly take aspirin. There was no association between fish or omega-3 poly-unsaturated fatty acid intake and risk of haemorrhagic stroke. These findings indicate that higher consumption of fish and omega-3 polyunsaturated fatty acids is associated with a reduced risk of thrombotic infarction, primarily among women who do not take aspirin regularly, but is not related to risk of haemorrhagic stroke.

5.8   Milk consumption

An association between milk consumption and reduced risk of ischaemic stroke in older middle-aged men, which could not be explained by intake of dietary calcium, has been reported (Abbott et al. 1996).

5.9   Obesity

Obesity has been found to have an independent relation to CHD, but evidence for an association between general obesity and risk of stroke is weak. Abbott et al. (1994) studied 1163 non-smoking men of mean age 55–65 years and followed them up for 22 years. They reported that elevated body mass index was associated with an increased risk of thromboembolic stroke in non-smoking men in older middle age who are free of commonly observed conditions related to cardiovascular disease. In a study of 28 643 US male health professionals aged 40–75 years having no history of stroke, Walker et al. (1996) found during 5 years of follow-up that abdominal obesity, but not elevated BMI, predicts risk of stroke. In another study from the USA, more than 12 000 adults aged 45–64 years, having no cardiovascular disease at baseline, had their diabetic status measured using fasting glucose criteria, waist and hip circumference and fasting insulin levels. During 6–8 years of follow-up, diabetes was found to be a strong risk factor for ischaemic stroke occurrence. Insulin resistance, as reflected by waist to hip ratios and elevated fasting insulin levels, may also contribute to a greater risk of ischaemic stroke (Folsom et al. 1999).

5.10   Physical activity

Regular exercise has well established benefits for reducing the risk of premature death and other cardiovascular disease (Gorelick et al. 1999). The beneficial effect of lowering the risk of stroke has been described predominately among whites, is more apparent for men than women, and younger rather than older adults (Fletcher 1994). A dose–response relationship between increasing amounts of physical activity and the reduction in the risk of stroke has not been shown consistently. The protective effect of physical activity may be partly mediated through its role in controlling various risk factors for stroke (e.g. hypertension, diabetes and obesity) by accompanying reductions in plasma fibrinogen levels and platelet activity, and elevation in plasma tissue plasminogen activator activity and high density lipoprotein concentrations (Manson et al. 1991; Lakka & Salonen 1993; Kokkinos et al. 1995; Rangemark et al. 1995; Wang et al. 1995; Blair et al. 1996; Williams 1996).

Recently, the association between physical activity and risk of total stroke and stroke sub-types in women has been examined in the prospective cohort Nurses' Health Study in the USA: 72 488 female nurses aged 40 to 65 years, who did not have diagnosed cardiovascular disease or cancer at baseline in 1986, completed detailed physical activity questionnaires in 1986, 1988 and 1992. The results showed that physical activity, including moderate-intensity exercise such as walking, is associated in a dose–response manner with a substantial reduction in the risk of total and ischaemic stroke (Hu et al. 2000). Another study by Hu et al. (2001) examined whether physical activity decreases risk for cardiovascular disease among diabetic women; after adjustment for smoking, BMI and other cardiovascular risk factors, it was found that increased physical activity, including regular walking, was associated with substantially reduced risk for cardiovascular events including ischaemic strokes.

5.11 Alcohol use

Alcohol consumption may have a direct dose-dependent effect on the risk of haemorrhagic stroke (Donahue et al. 1986). For cerebral infarction, results have ranged from a definite independent effect in both men and women, an effect only in men, and no effect after controlling for other confounding risk factors such as cigarette smoking (Gorelick 1989). A J-shaped relationship between alcohol use and ischaemic stroke has been proposed, with a protective effect in light or moderate drinkers and an elevated stroke risk with heavy alcohol consumption (Gill et al. 1986). Alcohol may increase the risk of stroke through various mechanisms, including induction of hypertension, hypercoagulable states, cardiac arrhythmias and cerebral blood flow reductions. There is evidence that light to moderate drinking may have beneficial effects by increasing HDL cholesterol levels and decreasing platelet aggregation and fibrinogen levels (Thornton et al. 1983; Pellegrini et al. 1996; Gorelick et al. 1999). In 1998, The American Heart Association published recommendations for alcohol consumption: moderate consumption of alcohol may prevent atherosclerotic heart disease, but heavy use of alcohol should be avoided (Biller et al. 1998).

5.12   Maternal and fetal nutrition

Maternal nutrition is now thought to have an important influence on rates of cardiovascular diseases and their related risk factors in the next generation. The findings of an ecological study in London showing that healthy and well nourished mothers in London at the beginning of the twentieth century had children who now have low death rates from ischaemic heart disease and stroke support this view (Barker et al. 1992). Recent findings also suggest that many human fetuses have to adapt to a limited supply of nutrients and in doing so permanently change their physiology and metabolism; these 'programmed' changes may be the origins of a number of diseases in later life, including IHD and related disorders such as stroke, diabetes and hypertension (Barker 1997). However, the true impact of maternal nutrition on fetal development and risk of disease in later life is not yet known, and there is a need for further independent epidemiological, animal and clinical studies.

5.13   Genetic and racial factors

Many diet-related chronic diseases, such as diabetes, hypertension, stroke, IHD and cancer, are more common among some ethnic groups than among white people (Bertron et al. 1999). For example, Qureshi et al. (1999) reported that African Americans have double the risk of intracerebral haemorrhage than white Americans, most of which may be explained by racial differences in systolic blood pressure and low educational attainment which is also a risk factor for cigarette smoking and development of hypertension, obesity and high cholesterol levels. Nutritional factors may have an important role to play in increased risk of stroke among ethnically and genetically different groups; however, this increased risk is more likely to be the result of complex interactions between socio-economic status, physical inactivity, limited access to health care, and genetic and environmental factors.

5.14   Summary

Observational studies support the role of modifying lifestyle-related risk factors such as diet, physical activity and alcohol use in stroke prevention. For example, increased sodium intake is associated with hypertension, and reduction in salt consumption may significantly lower blood pressure and reduce stroke mortality. Moderately elevated homocysteine levels may be associated with stroke and are associated with insufficient dietary intake of folate, vitamins B6 and B12. Consumption of a diet rich in fruits, vegetables, folate, potassium, calcium, magnesium, fibre, fish and milk may protect against stroke. Regular physical activity may also protect against stroke through its role in controlling various risk factors such as hypertension, diabetes mellitus and obesity. The role of fat intake as a risk factor for stroke remains uncertain, whereas the association between stroke and cholesterol level has more convincingly been demonstrated by recent intervention trials using statins. There is also evidence that low serum albumin levels may be causally linked to stroke risk and outcome.

6 Antioxidants and Risk of Ischaemic Stroke

6.1 Introduction

There are several reasons why increased consumption of fruit and vegetables is desirable in the diet. They are a rich source of non-starch polysaccharides and vitamins and minerals; several of these micronutrients have antioxidant properties and may have a role in protecting against free radical-induced oxidative stress which has been linked with the pathogenesis of ischaemic stroke and ischaemic heart disease (IHD) and other diseases (Gey et al. 1993a). These essential antioxidants include vitamins C, E, A and carotenoids, and their concentration in body fluids is determined mainly by dietary intake (Gey et al. 1993a).

Table 6.1 lists some recent epidemiological studies regarding the association between antioxidants and incidence of ischaemic stroke. In Great Britain, for example, rates of strokes and IHD are highest in regions where consumption of fruit and vegetables is lowest, and an inverse association between fruit and vegetable consumption and incidence of stroke was suggested (Acheson & Williams 1983). Many epidemiological studies from all over the world have indicated that vegetable-rich diets are associated with a higher life expectancy; antioxidants could be of principal importance in conferring the benefits of vegetable-rich diets.

6.2 Intake of antioxidant vitamins and risk of cardiovascular disease

There is a substantial body of epidemiological evidence linking intake of antioxidant vitamins, particularly vitamin E, with reduced risk of coronary disease (Brown & Hu 2001). There are three major epidemiological complementary studies of the relationship between the plasma concentration of diet-derived antioxidants and the risk of IHD and stroke:

(1) The WHO MONICA (World Health Organization 1989) which was a cross-cultural comparison of randomly selected representatives of 16 European study populations.
(2) The Edinburgh Angina-Control Study (Riemersma et al. 1991) which was

Table 6.1 Epidemiological trials of association between fruit and vegetable (antioxidant) intake and incidence of stroke

Authors & country	Participants	Sample size	Age (years)	Length of follow-up (years)	Antioxidants	End-points	Comments
Basel Prospective Study (Gey et al. 1993b); Switzerland	Volunteering men of the working population	2974	50 ± 9	12	Plasma carotene and vitamin C	31 incident strokes	Increased incidence of stroke at low concentration of both vitamin C and plasma carotene (risk adjusted for age, smoking, blood pressure and cholesterol)
Manson et al. 1993; USA	Female nurses free of diagnosed IHD and cancer at baseline (1980)	87 245	34–59	8	Dietary carotene and vitamins C & E	183 incident strokes	After adjustment for age, smoking and other cardiovascular risk factors, higher antioxidant vitamin consumption (all three) is associated with a reduced risk of ischaemic stroke
Gale et al. 1995; UK	Randomly selected elderly people (1973–1974) free of history or symptoms of stroke or IHD living in the community	730	65 and over	20	Dietary and plasma vitamin C	643 died (124 because of stroke)	Mortality from stroke was highest in those who had the lowest vitamin C levels; low vitamin C whether measured by plasma concentration or dietary intake, was strongly related to subsequent risk of death from stroke but not from IHD
Gillman et al. 1995; USA	Framingham population-based longitudinal study. Men free of cardiovascular disease at baseline (1966–1969)	832	45–65	> 20	Estimated from servings per day of fruits and vegetables from a single 24-hour diet recall at baseline	97 incident strokes (73 complete strokes and 24 transient ischaemic attacks)	The risk of complete stroke or transient ischaemic attack was adjusted for BMI, cigarette smoking, glucose intolerance, physical activity, blood pressure, serum cholesterol, and energy, ethanol and fat intake. There was an inverse association between fruit and vegetable intake and the development of stroke; the intake of fruit and vegetables may protect against development of stroke in men

Reference	Population	n	Age	Years	Exposure	Outcome	Findings
Keli et al. 1996 The Netherlands	Randomly selected men free of stroke from the town of Zutphen (1960)	552	50–69	15	Dietary history taken in 1960, 1965 and 1970	42 incident strokes	After adjusting for age, systolic blood pressure, serum cholesterol, smoking, energy intake and consumption of fish and alcohol, dietary flavonoids (quercetin) and β-carotene intake were inversely associated with stroke incidence; intake of vitamins C and E was not associated with stroke risk
Khaw & Barrett-Connor 1987; USA	A 30% sub-sample of a defined upper-middle class white community in Rancho Bernardo, CA, who participated in a survey of risk factors for heart disease	859	50–79	12	24-hour dietary potassium intake at baseline	24 died of stroke	Inverse association of potassium intake, irrespective of hypertensive status, with stroke mortality; high dietary intake of potassium may protect against stroke-associated death
Lui et al. 2000; USA	Women free of diagnosed IHD, stroke and diabetes mellitus in 1984	75 521	38–63	12	Dietary wholegrain intake	352 incident strokes	After adjustment for age, smoking and other risk factors, higher wholegrain intake is associated with a reduced risk of ischaemic stroke

a case-control study of 110 undiagnosed and untreated angina pectoris sufferers and 394 matched controls identified by mail questionnaires from 600 males.

(3)   The Basel Prospective Study (Gey et al. 1993b) of 2974 volunteer men from the working population aged 50 ± 9 years.

These studies consistently revealed an increased risk of IHD (and stroke) at low plasma concentrations of antioxidants. During 12 years follow-up of the Basel Prospective Study, 132 subjects died of IHD and 31 of stroke. Subjects with low concentrations of both carotene and vitamin C had a significantly higher risk of death from these conditions. Manson et al. (1993) assessed consumption of antioxidant vitamins using a semiquantitative food frequency questionnaire of 87 245 US female nurses aged 34 to 59 years; participants who were free of diagnosed IHD and cancer were followed up for 8 years. They found that high antioxidant vitamin consumption was associated with a reduced risk of ischaemic stroke in women. In the same cohort, Stampfer et al. (1993) reported that the relative risk (RR) of IHD was 0.66 (95% CI, 0.50–0.87) for women in the highest quintile of vitamin E intake compared with those in the lowest quintile. A similar reduction in risk was observed in the Health Professionals' Follow-Up Study (Rimm et al. 1993). Knekt et al. (1994) reported an inverse association between dietary vitamin E intake and coronary mortality in both healthy men (RR for extreme tertiles, 0.68; 95% CI, 0.42–1.11) and women (RR, 0.34; 95% CI, 0.14–0.88). The Iowa Women's Study found that dietary vitamin E intake, as opposed to supplemental vitamin E, was inversely associated with the risk of death from IHD (Kushi et al. 1996). An additional study by Losonczy et al. (1996), in an elderly population, showed a reduced risk of all-cause mortality and CHD mortality with increased vitamin E intake (including both supplements and diet); these authors also found that supplementation with both vitamin E and vitamin C further reduced the risk of total and coronary mortality, suggesting a synergistic effect of vitamins E and C. Prospective cohort studies on the relationship between vitamin C and cardiovascular disease (CVD) are limited and inconsistent. Neither the Nurses' Health Study nor the Health Professionals' Follow-Up Study found a significant association between vitamin C consumption and risk of CHD. However, the First National Health and Nutrition Examination Survey epidemiological follow-up study found that higher vitamin C intake was associated with a reduced risk of total mortality in men and of cardiovascular death in men and women (Enstrom et al. 1992).

The results of a number of clinical trials have been published regarding the effects of vitamin E supplementation on the risk of CVD: the Cambridge Heart Antioxidant Study (CHAOS) (Stephens et al. 1996), the Alpha-Tocopherol, Beta-Carotene Cancer Prevention Study (ATBC) (Alpha-Tocopherol, Beta-Carotene Cancer Prevention Study Group 1994), the GISSI-Prevenzione trial

(GISSI-Prevenzione Investigators 1999), the Heart Outcomes Prevention Evaluation (HOPE) Study (Yusuf et al. 2000) and the MRC/BHF Heart Protection Study (Heart Protection Study Collaborative Group 2002). CHAOS enrolled 2002 patients with documented CVD and evaluated daily supplementation with 400 or 800 IU of tocopherol. The treatment resulted in a RR of 0.53 (95% CI, 0.34–0.83) for cardiovascular death and non-fatal myocardial infarction, the decreased risk being due predominantly to the reduction in non-fatal myocardial infarction in the treatment group. The ATBC trial assessed daily supplementation with 50 mg (75 IU) of vitamin E or 20 mg β-carotene, or both, on cardiovascular outcomes in 27 271 male smokers. The trial reported a non-significant, small reduction in the incidence of fatal coronary disease, but was considered to have used too low a dose of tocopherol. The ATBC investigators recently reported that there was no effect on intermittent claudication either (Tornwall et al. 1999). The GISSI-Prevenzione trial studied 3658 patients with a previous myocardial infarction and assessed the effect of daily supplementation with 300 mg vitamin E on cardiovascular outcomes. Although there was no significant effect of vitamin E on the combined end-points of cardiovascular death, non-fatal myocardial infarction and non-fatal stroke (RR, 0.88; 95% CI, 0.75–1.04), there appeared to be a significantly decreased risk of cardiovascular death, including cardiac, coronary and sudden death (RR, 0.80; 95% CI, 0.65–0.99). Finally, the HOPE study, which enrolled 2545 women and 6996 men with a high risk of CVD (existing CVD or diabetes), showed that supplementation with 400 IU vitamin E daily had no effect on cardiovascular outcomes in this population over a period of 4.5 years; the RR was 1.05 (95% CI, 0.95–1.16) for primary outcomes (myocardial infarction, stroke and death from cardiovascular causes).

6.3   Intake of antioxidant vitamins and risk of stroke

Two large cohort follow-up studies reported in 1995; that from the UK was a 20 year follow-up of 730 randomly selected elderly people free of history or symptoms of stroke or IHD and living in the community. They all had their vitamin C status assessed by dietary intake and plasma concentration. During the 20 years of follow-up, 643 subjects died, 124 of these from stroke. Mortality from stroke was highest in those who had the lowest vitamin C levels; low vitamin C level, whether measured by plasma concentration or dietary intake, was strongly related to subsequent risk of death from stroke but not from IHD (Gale et al. 1995).

The other study was part of the Framingham population-based longitudinal study in which the diet of 832 men, aged 45 to 65 years, was assessed by a single 24-hour recall, and subjects were followed up for 20 years. The risk of completed stroke or transient ischaemic attack was adjusted for BMI, cigarette smoking, glucose intolerance, physical activity, blood pressure, serum cholesterol, and energy, ethanol and fat intake. There was an inverse association between fruit and vegetable intake and the development of stroke, however, and the authors concluded that the intake of fruit and vegetables might protect against development of stroke in men (Gillman et al. 1995). Habitual intake of flavonoids and their major source (tea) may also protect against stroke (Keli et al. 1996).

In contrast, a small hospital-based study in which the dietary and plasma vitamin C status was assessed in a non-randomly selected group of patients with a high probability of cerebral thrombosis and within 5-year age matched controls failed to demonstrate a relationship between vitamin C status and the risk of stroke (Barer et al. 1989). A randomised intervention trial in 22071 male doctors aged 40 to 84 years found that β-carotene had no effect on incidences of cancer, CVD and stroke after 14 years of follow-up (Hennekens et al. 1996). Three large, randomised, double-blind intervention trials using vitamin E have reported outcome data on stroke but were all negative (Table 6.2). Of these, the HOPE trial (Yusuf et al. 2000) used 400 IU of vitamin E daily and an angiotensin-converting enzyme inhibitor (ramapril) in a 2 × 2 factorial design. The average age of the patients was 66 years; a little over half had had a previous myocardial infarction and approximately one-quarter had unstable angina. The end-point was a composite of non-fatal infarction, stroke or death from cardiovascular causes. Vitamin E had no effect on stroke. The GISSI trial (GISSI-Prevenzione Investigators 1999) compared synthetic vitamin E (300 mg daily) and omega-3 polyunsaturated fatty acids (1 g daily) in a 2 × 2 factorial design. The patients all had a myocardial infarction within 3 months of being randomised. Over a 3.5-year follow-up, vitamin E had no effect on the composite end-point of death, non-fatal myocardial infarction and stroke.

Very recently, the Heart Protection Study Collaborative Group (2002) studied the relationship between increased intake of antioxidant vitamins and incidence of vascular disease including stroke in 20 536 UK adults (aged 40–80 years) with coronary disease, other occlusive arterial disease or diabetes. Subjects were randomly allocated to receive daily antioxidant vitamin supplementation (600 mg vitamin E, 250 mg vitamin C and 20 mg β-carotene) or matching placebo. Intention-to-treat comparisons of outcome were conducted between all vitamin-allocated and all placebo-allocated participants. An average of 83% of participants in each treatment group remained compliant during the scheduled 5-year treatment period. Allocation to this vitamin regimen approximately doubled the plasma concentration of α-tocopherol, increased that of vitamin C by one-third, and quadrupled that of β-carotene. Primary outcomes were major coronary events (for overall analyses) and fatal or non-fatal vascular events (for subcategory analyses), with subsidiary assessments of cancer and of other major morbidity. There were no significant differences in all-cause mortality in vitamin-allocated versus placebo-

Table 6.2 Randomised controlled trials of supplementation with antioxidants and risk of stroke

Authors & country	Participants	Sample size	Age (years)	Length of follow-up (years)	Antioxidant supplements	End-point	Comments
Hennekens et al. 1996; USA	Randomised, double-blind, placebo-controlled trial of male physicians (11% current smokers & 39% former smokers at the beginning of the study)	22071	40–84	12	50 mg of β-carotene on alternate days	Maliganant neoplasm, myocardial infarction or stroke	Neither benefit nor harm in terms of the incidence of malignant disease, myocardial infarction or stroke
GISSI Trial 1999; Italy	Patients surviving recent myocardial infarction (≤ 3 months)	11324	59	3.5 yrs	A daily 300 mg vitamin E, 1 g n-3 PUFA,[a] both or neither	Death, non-fatal myocardial infarction infarction and stroke	Dietary supplementation with n-3 PUFA led to a clinically important and significant benefit; vitamin E had no benefit
HOPE Trial (Yusuf et al. 2000); USA	Men and women who had cardiovascular disease or diabetes in addition to one other risk factor	2545 women + 6996 men	55 or older	4.5 years	400 IU of vitamin E daily or matching placebo, and ramipril or matching placebo	Myocardial infarction, stroke and death from cardiovascular causes	Vitamin E had no apparent effect on cardiovascular outcomes
Heart Protection Study Collaborative Group 2002; UK	UK adults with coronary disease, other occlusive arterial disease, or diabetes	20536	40–80	5 years	600 mg vitamin E, 250 mg vitamin C, and 20 mg β-carotene daily or events placebo	Coronary events, and fatal or non-fatal vascular events	Although the antioxidant vitamins were safe and increased blood vitamin concentrations substantially, they did not produce any significant reductions in mortality or incidence of any type of vascular disease

[a] n-3 Polyunsaturated fatty acid.

allocated, or in deaths due to vascular or non-vascular causes; nor were there any significant differences in the numbers of participants having non-fatal myocardial infarction or coronary death, non-fatal or fatal stroke, or coronary or non-coronary revascularisation. There were also no significant effects on cancer incidence or on hospitalisation for any other non-vascular cause. Among the high-risk individuals who were studied, these antioxidant vitamins appeared to be safe. However, although this regimen increased blood vitamin concentrations substantially, it did not produce any significant reductions in the 5-year mortality from, or incidence of, any type of vascular disease, cancer, or other major outcome.

A prospective cohort study that has examined the association between antioxidant vitamin intakes and death from stroke in a cohort of 34 492 post-menopausal women, reported 215 deaths from stroke during follow-up. The results suggested a protective effect of vitamin E from foods on death from stroke, but did not support a protective role for supplemental vitamin E or other antioxidant vitamins. However, given the number of deaths from stroke in the cohort, a small-to-moderate association could not be ruled out (Yochum et al. 2000).

Although increased intake of grain products has been recommended to prevent cardiovascular disease, prospective data examining the relationship between whole grain intake and risk of ischaemic stroke are sparse. Liu et al. (2000) examined the relationship between whole grain intake and risk of ischaemic stroke in a prospective cohort of 75 521 US women aged 38 to 63 years without previous diagnosis of diabetes mellitus, CHD, stroke, or other CVDs in 1984, who completed detailed food frequency questionnaires in 1984, 1986, 1990 and 1994, and were followed up for 12 years as part of the Nurses' Health Study. Their main outcome measures were incidence of ischaemic stroke, confirmed by medical records, by quintile of whole grain intake according to questionnaire responses. During 861 900 person-years of follow-up, there were 352 confirmed ischaemic strokes. An inverse association between whole grain intake and ischaemic stroke risk was observed. The age-adjusted RRs from the lowest to highest quintiles of whole grain intake were 1.00 (referent), 0.68 (95% CI, 0.49–0.94), 0.69 (95% CI, 0.51–0.95), 0.49 (95% CI, 0.35–0.69) and 0.57 (95% CI, 0.42–0.78; $P = 0.003$ for trend). Adjustment for smoking modestly attenuated this association (RR comparing extreme quintiles, 0.64; 95% CI, 0.47–0.89). This inverse association remained essentially unchanged with further adjustment for known CVD risk factors, including saturated fat and *trans* fatty acid intake (multivariate-adjusted RR comparing extreme quintiles, 0.69; 95% CI, 0.50–0.98). An inverse relationship between whole grain intake and risk of ischaemic stroke was also consistently observed among sub-groups of women who never smoked, did not drink alcohol, did not exercise regularly, or who did not use post-menopausal hormones. In this cohort of women, higher intake of whole grain foods was found to be associated with a lower risk of ischaemic stroke, independent of known CVD risk factors, supporting the notion that higher intake of whole grains may reduce the risk of ischaemic stroke.

6.4 Interpretation of results

The reasons for the quite different results between the CHAOS and the GISSI and HOPE trials remain unknown, despite the large number of cases studied in the GISSI and HOPE trials (a total of 7991 randomised to vitamin E). Halliwell's (2000) explanation for this paradox is that antioxidants are reducing agents which act by scavenging damaging oxidising agents such as free radicals. Transition metal ions, released as a result of injury by oxidative damage, act as catalysts of free radical damage, especially in the reduced state. If, for example, a powerful antioxidant (i.e. a powerful reducing agent) is administered after oxidative damage has started, it could promote damage (i.e. be pro-oxidant); in this situation, the more powerful the antioxidant, the more problems it might cause. Therefore administration of antioxidants can give protective effects or worsen damage, depending on where they act in the sequence of events.

In his review, Steinberg (2000) reported that *in vitro* and animal model studies provide both direct and indirect evidence that oxidation of low-density lipoprotein and/or related oxidative mechanisms play a role in atherogenesis. However, the HOPE and GISSI clinical intervention trials unexpectedly gave negative results, possibly because the animal intervention evidence on which they were based deals primarily with very early lesions (fatty streaks); such evidence does not necessarily provide a basis for predicting what antioxidant intervention will do in patients with advanced lesions, particularly when the end-points used relate to unstable plaques and fatal thrombosis, events for which we have no adequate animal models. Nor does it necessarily follow that the same antioxidants used successfully in animals will be effective in humans. The strength of the evidence for the oxidative modification hypothesis is such that negative clinical trials lasting only 3–5 years, with one particular antioxidant in patients with very advanced CHD, should not be taken as refutation of the hypothesis. Perhaps different human trials are needed in which the development of new lesions is measured, to test whether antioxidants can decrease the rate of initiation and early progression of atherosclerosis as they do in animals.

The overall results of the clinical trials are somewhat disappointing given the consistent and promising findings from epidemiological studies. However, more conclusive evidence may be forthcoming from several on-going clinical trials.

6.5 Summary

Many epidemiological studies from all over the world have led to the assumption that vegetable-rich diets are associated with a higher life expectancy, and antioxidants could be of principal importance in conferring the benefits of vegetable-rich diets. With regard to the use of antioxidants for the treatment of human disease, such as coronary heart disease and stroke, there have been some contradictory results; there are, however, several on-going clinical trials which should help to provide more conclusive evidence.

There is strong indirect evidence that antioxidants may protect against free radical-induced oxidative stress, which has been linked to the pathogenesis of ischaemic stroke. The neuroprotective effect of antioxidants is not definitely established and needs to be studied further. However, the administration of antioxidants can give protective effects or worsen damage, depending on where they act in the sequence of events.

7 Homocysteine and Stroke

7.1 Introduction

The homocysteine theory of atherosclerosis was based originally on the presence of cardiovascular disease in those with inborn errors of homocysteine metabolism (McCully 1969). Although several case-control and prospective cohort studies showed associations between modest elevation of total plasma homocysteine and cardiovascular disease (CVD), including stroke, it is only relatively recently that sufficient evidence has accumulated to suggest that the association is independent and dose-related (Hankey & Eikelboom 1999).

Several observations suggest that homocysteine has a role in the development of vascular diseases. For example, homocysteine may promote the oxidation of low-density lipoprotein (LDL) cholesterol, vascular smooth muscle cell proliferation, activation of platelet and coagulation factors and endothelial dysfunction (Heinecke et al. 1993; Demuth et al. 1999; Holven et al. 2001).

The prevalence of hyperhomocysteinaemia in the general population is between 5% and 10%; however, rates may be as high as 30% to 40% in the elderly population (Selhub et al. 1993). Homocysteine may, therefore, represent an important and potentially modifiable risk factor for stroke.

7.2 Homocysteine metabolism

Homocysteine is a sulphydryl-containing amino acid derived from the metabolic demethylation of dietary methionine, which is abundant in animal protein. It is present in plasma in four forms: about 1% circulates as the free thiol; 70–80% is disulphide-bound to plasma proteins, chiefly albumin; and the remaining 20–30% combines with itself to form the dimer homocysteine or with other thiols, including cysteine, with which it forms the homocysteine–cysteine mixed disulphide (Ueland 1995). The term 'total plasma (or serum) homocysteine' refers to the combined pool of all four forms of homocysteine. Homocysteine is metabolised by remethylation or *trans*-sulphuration (Figure 7.1).

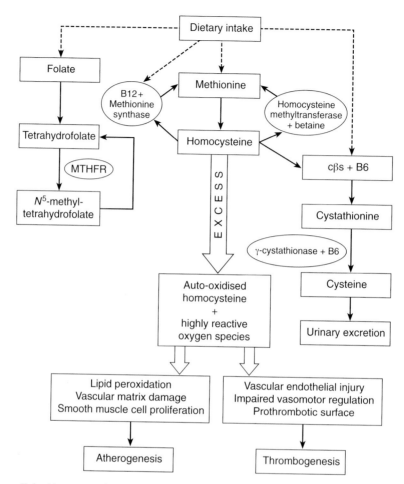

Figure 7.1 Homocysteine metabolism and possible mechanism of atherothrombotic disease. Reproduced from Hankey & Eikelboom (1999) with permission of Elsevier Science.

7.2.1   Remethylation

Under conditions of low protein intake, homocysteine is metabolised primarily via one of two methionine-conserving remethylation pathways (Finkelstein 1998). In the liver, a substantial proportion of homocysteine is remethylated by betaine–homocysteine methyltransferase with betaine as the methyl donor. In most other tissues, the remethylation is catalysed by methionine synthase with N^5-methyltetrahydrofolate as the donor. The formation of this methyl donor depends on the presence of N^5,N^{10}-methylene-tetrahydrofolate (derived from dietary folate) and the enzyme N^5,N^{10}-

methylenetetrahydrofolate reductase (MTHFR). Vitamin B12 (cobalamin) is an essential cofactor for methionine synthase (Finkelstein 1998).

7.2.2   Trans-sulphuration

When the remethylation pathway is saturated, or when cysteine is required, homocysteine is converted to cystathionine (and then cysteine) by cystathionine β-synthase (CβS) (Finkelstein 1998); vitamin B6 (pyridoxine) is an essential cofactor. Cysteine may be metabolised further to sulphate and excreted in the urine (Finkelstein 1998).

7.3   Factors influencing homocysteine metabolism (Table 7.1)

These can be placed into three main groups:

- Genetic defects
- Nutritional deficiencies
- Other causes, such as renal impairment, vascular disease or drug side-effects.

Table 7.1   Factors increasing plasma homocysteine levels (from Hankey & Eikelboom (1999), reprinted with permission from Elsevier Science).

Genetic defects in homocysteine metabolism
- CβS
- MTHFR
- Methionine synthase

Nutritional deficiencies in vitamin cofactors
- Folate
- Vitamin B12 (cobalamin)
- Vitamin B6 (pyridoxine)

Diseases
- Pernicious anaemia
- Renal impairment
- Hypothyroidism
- Malignancy: acute lymphoblastic leukaemia, carcinoma of the breast, ovary and pancreas
- Severe psoriasis

Medications/toxins
- Folate antagonists (methotrexate, phenytoin, carbamazepine)
- Vitamin B6 antagonists (theophylline, azarabine, oestrogen-containing oral contraceptives, cigarette smoking)

Age/sex
- Increasing age
- Male sex
- Menopause

7.3.1 Genetic defects

The most common of the genetic causes of severe hyperhomocysteinaemia and classic homocystinuria (congenital homocystinuria) is homozygous deficiency of CβS. It occurs in only one in 100 000 live births and results in an increase of up to 40-fold in fasting total plasma homocysteine. It is inherited as an autosomal recessive trait (Mudd et al. 1985). The heterozygous form (about one in 150 of the population) is often associated with normal basal plasma total homocysteine, and it is uncertain whether heterozygosity is associated with additional risk of vascular events (Hankey & Eikelboom 1999).

The most common enzyme defect associated with moderately raised total homocysteine is a point mutation (C to T substitution at nucleotide 677) in the coding region of the gene for MTHFR, which is associated with a thermolabile MTHFR variant that has about half-normal activity (Kang et al. 1988). 10–13% of white populations are homozygous for this mutation (TT genotype) (Frosst et al. 1995) and in the presence of a suboptimal folate intake will have a moderately raised (by about 50%) total plasma homocysteine level (Malinow et al. 1997).

7.3.2 Nutritional deficiencies

Because blood levels of folate, vitamin B12 and, to a lesser extent, vitamin B6 are related inversely to hyperhomocysteinaemia (Selhub et al. 1993), anyone with a nutritional deficiency that leads to low blood concentrations of folate, vitamin B12 or vitamin B6 is at increased risk of hyperhomocysteinaemia (Kang et al. 1987). Indeed, it has been suggested that about two-thirds of cases of hyperhomocysteinaemia are due to inadequate blood levels of one or more of these vitamin cofactors (Selhub et al. 1993).

7.3.3 Other causes

Renal impairment commonly causes hyperhomocysteinaemia. Fasting total homocysteine rises as serum creatinine rises, not because of impaired urinary excretion but because of impaired metabolism of homocysteine by the kidney, the major route by which homocysteine is cleared from plasma (Bostom & Lathrop 1997; Hankey & Eikelboom 1999). Total homocysteine levels are considerably higher in patients with chronic renal disease than the moderately raised concentrations commonly found in patients with atherothrombotic vascular disease, and this may contribute to the high incidence of vascular complications in patients with chronic renal failure. Plasma homocysteine concentrations can be increased by various drugs and diseases that interfere with folate, vitamin B6 and vitamin B12 metabolism, and an abnormal homocysteine concentration may therefore be used as a diagnostic aid for some of these conditions (Savage et al. 1994).

7.4   Measurement of plasma homocysteine

The most robust measure is total homocysteine, which is assumed to represent biologically active homocysteine, directly or indirectly (Ueland 1995). The most widely used method is high performance liquid chromatography (Still & McDowell 1998), but other simple, reliable and inexpensive methods are available (Frantzen et al. 1998). The measurement can be done fasting or non-fasting, and before and after oral methionine loading; Hankey and Eikelboom (1999) recommend that total homocysteine be measured after fasting for at least 12 h, to avoid the variable rise that may occur after a meal (Guttormsen et al. 1994).

7.5   Prevalence of hyperhomocysteinaemia

The prevalence of hyperhomocysteinaemia has been estimated to be 5% in the general population, and 13–47% among patients with symptomatic athero-sclerotic vascular disease (McCully 1996; Malinow et al. 1998); however, these estimates are based on a cut-off above the 90th or 95th percentile of the distribution of total homocysteine in the general population. Hankey and Eikelboom (1999) recommend that hyperhomocysteinaemia be defined as a plasma level of total homocysteine that correlates with an increased risk of atherosclerotic vascular events. However, there is no definite threshold that correlates with a sudden increase in the risk of vascular events; indeed, the relation between total homocysteine and risk appears to be linear (or log-linear), in much the same way that increasing blood pressure and cholesterol are related to vascular disease (Hankey & Eikelboom 1999).

7.6   Association between hyperhomocysteinaemia and vascular damage

The mechanism by which homocysteine might cause vascular damage is unclear. Experimental evidence suggests that homocysteine promotes athero-genesis by facilitating oxidative arterial injury, damaging the vascular matrix and augmenting the proliferation of vascular smooth muscle. It may promote thromboembolic disease by causing oxidative injury to the endothelium, altering the coagulant properties of the blood and impairing endothelium-dependent vasomotor regulation (Figure 7.1) (Welch et al. 1997). However, most *in vitro* and volunteer studies have been done with homocysteine concentrations at least ten times greater than those seen in patients with moderate hyperhomocysteinaemia, and should therefore be interpreted with caution. An atherogenic and/or prothrombotic effect of homocysteine remains unproven (Hankey & Eikelboom 1999).

7.7   Homocysteine and atherothrombotic vascular disease

There is now strong evidence of increased risk of atherosclerosis in subjects with mild to moderate elevation of total plasma homocysteine compared with controls (Brattstrom & Wilcken 2000; Ueland et al. 2000). Homocysteine concentrations are elevated in up to 30% of patients with atherosclerosis (Clarke et al. 1991), and levels only 12% above the upper limit of normal (15 µmol/l, mild hyperhomocysteinaemia), are associated with a threefold increase in the risk of vascular events, including strokes (Nygard et al. 1997). Atherosclerosis leading to these events is characterised by a thickening of the arterial wall due to smooth muscle cell proliferation, lipid deposits and fibrosis (Davies 1995).

The epidemiological evidence that links increasing homocysteine with an increasing risk of atherothrombotic disease comes from the large prospective observational cohort studies of Stampfer et al. (1992), Alfthan et al. (1994), Verhoef et al. (1994, 1997), Arnesen et al. (1995), Perry et al. (1995), Chasan-Taber et al. (1996), Evans et al. (1997), Nygard et al. (1997), Folsom et al. (1998), Wald et al. (1998) (Table 7.2). A strong graded relation has been reported between increasing total homocysteine and overall mortality in individuals with angiographically demonstrated CHD (Nygard et al. 1997). However, other prospective studies, including further reports from the Physicians' Health Study, have not found a significant association between hyperhomocysteinaemia and myocardial infarction or stroke (Hankey & Eikelboom 1999). In 1995, Boushey et al. reported a meta-analysis of 27 observational studies (23 cross-sectional or retrospective case-control and four-nested case-control studies based on prospective cohorts), including about 4000 patients. A raised total homocysteine (usually defined as above the 90th or 95th percentile of controls) was associated with an increased risk of fatal and non-fatal atherosclerotic vascular disease in the coronary (odds ratio (OR), 1.7; 95% CI, 1.5–1.9), cerebral (OR, 2.5; CI, 2.0–3.0) and peripheral (OR, 6.8; CI, 2.9–15.8) circulations. The magnitude of risk was similar to that for other risk factors, such as hypercholesterolaemia and smoking, and it was estimated that about 10% of CHD in the general population might be attributable to elevated homocysteine levels (Boushey et al. 1995). From an analysis that assumed a graded, linear relation between homocysteine levels and vascular risk, Boushey et al. (1995) also estimated that a 5 µmol/l increase in total homocysteine was associated

Table 7.2 Homocysteine and cardiovascular risk, prospective cohort and nested case-control studies. (Adapted from Hankey & Eikelboom (1999) with permission from Elsevier Science).

Study	Sex	Cases/controls	Major end-points[a]	Total homocysteine		Relative risk (95% CI)
				Cases	Controls	
Physicians' Health Study, USA (Stampfer et al. 1992)	M	271/27	Fatal/non-fatal MI and CHD death	11.1	10.5	3.4 (1.3–8.8)
BUPA, UK (Wald et al. 1998)	M	229/1126	Fatal CHD	≥ 15.2	< 10.3	2.9 (2.04–4.1)
Tromso, Norway (Arnesen et al. 1995)	M/F	123/492	Fatal/non-fatal CHD	12.7	11.3	1.32 (1.05–1.65)
British Regional Heart Study (Perry et al. 1995)	M	107/118	Fatal/non-fatal stroke	13.7	11.9	2.8 (1.3–5.9)
Belgium (Nygard et al. 1997)	M/F	64 cases only	Death	≥ 20	≤ 9.0	4.5 (1.22–16.6)
Physicians' Health Study, USA (Chasan-Taber et al. 1996)	M	333/333	Fatal/non-fatal MI and CHD death	–	–	1.7 (0.9–3.3)
Physicians' Health Study, USA (Verhoef et al. 1997)	M	149/149	New angina, CABG	10.9	10.4	1.0 (0.4–2.4)
Physicians' Health Study, USA (Verhoef et al. 1994)	M	109/427	Ischaemic stroke	11.4	10.6	1.2 (0.7–2.0)
MRFIT, USA (Evans et al. 1997)	M M	93/186 147/286	Non-fatal MI CHD death	12.6 12.8	13.1 12.7	0.82 (0.55–54)
North Karelia Project, Finland (Alfthan et al. 1994)	M/F	265/269	Fatal/non-fatal MI, stroke	M 9.9 F 9.6	M 9.8 F 9.3	M 1.05 (0.56–1.95) F 1.22 (0.6–2.78)
ARIC, USA (Folsom et al. 1998)	M/F	232/537	Fatal/non-fatal MI	8.9	8.5	1.28 (0.5–3.2)

[a] CABG, coronary artery bypass graft; CAD, coronary artery disease; CHD, coronary heart disease; MI, myocardial infarction

with an increase in vascular risk of about one-third, which is of similar magnitude to an increase in plasma cholesterol of 0.5 mmol/l. The European Concerted Action Project also concluded that total homocysteine was an independent risk factor for atherosclerotic disease, and calculated that a 5 μmol/l increment in fasting basal total homocysteine was associated with relative risk (RR) of atherosclerotic vascular disease of 1.35 (1.1–1.6) in men and 1.42 (0.99–2.55) in women (Graham et al. 1997).

7.8   Homocysteine and stroke

Atherothrombotic vascular diseases are a common cause of stroke (Tortora & Grabowski 1996) as well as of CHD (Garrow et al. 2000). Only recently has sufficient evidence accumulated to suggest that the association of hyperhomocysteinaemia with vascular disease is independent and dose-related, but it remains to be established whether it is causal and modifiable. Many studies have reported an association between homocysteine levels and risk of stroke independent of other prognostic indicators (e.g. Perry et al. 1995; Giles et al. 1998).

Perry et al. (1995) examined the association between total serum homocysteine concentration and stroke in a case-control study. Between 1978 and 1980 serum was saved from 5661 British men with no history of stroke, aged 40–59 years, randomly selected from general practice; during follow-up to December 1991, there were 141 cases of stroke. Serum homocysteine was also measured in 118 control men matched for age group and town, without history of stroke at screening who did not develop stroke or myocardial infarction during follow-up. Homocysteine concentrations were significantly higher in stroke cases than controls. Perry et al. (1995) also reported a graded increase in relative risk of stroke in the second, third and fourth quarters of homocysteine distribution. Adjustment for some prognostic indicators did not attenuate the association, suggesting that homocysteine is a strong and independent risk factor for stroke. Giles et al. (1998) found in a nationally representative sample of black and white US adults ($n = 4534$) that high homocysteine concentration was independently associated with an increased likelihood of non-fatal stroke. High homocysteine levels may also be a risk factor for stroke in patients with sickle cell disease and systemic lupus erythematosus (Petri et al. 1996; Houston et al. 1997).

In contrast, Malinow et al. (1999) stated that although there is considerable epidemiological evidence for a relationship between plasma homocysteine and CVD, this has not been supported by all prospective studies. Moreover, despite the potential for reducing homocysteine levels with increased intake of folic acid, it is not known whether reduction of plasma homocysteine by diet and/or vitamin therapy will reduce CVD risk. Until results of controlled trials become available, population-wide screening is not recommended and emphasis should be placed on meeting current recommended daily allowances (RDAs) for folate and vitamins B6 and B12 by intake of vegetables, fruits, legumes, meats, fish, and fortified grains and cereals (Malinow et al. 1999).

There is some evidence that plasma total homocysteine concentrations may rise in a linear fashion within a 2-week period following acute ischaemic stroke (Howard et al. 2000). However, it is not known whether this rise is caused by the disease process itself, or if homocysteine is involved in an acute inflammatory response. There is a need to confirm this finding with larger studies.

High homocysteine levels may lead to endothelial damage (Harker et al. 1983; Matthias et al. 1996), affect platelet function and coagulation factors (Harker et al. 1976; Lentz et al. 1996;), and promote low density lipoprotein (LDL) oxidation (Heinecke et al. 1993). Increasing evidence suggests that homocysteine may exert these effects through an action on the endothelium. The association of homocysteine with endothelial dysfunction is reinforced by the fact that lowering plasma homocysteine with folic acid and pyridoxine may improve vascular function and nitric oxide-dependent vasodilation (Holven et al. 2001). *In vitro* studies suggest that homocysteine impairs endothelium-derived vasodilators (Demuth et al. 1999). Endothelial dysfunction in stroke will be discussed further in Chapter 8.

7.9   Intake of folic acid and other B-group vitamins and risk of cardiovascular disease

Folic acid, or folate, is a micronutrient found in many green leafy vegetables, such as spinach, and in some animal products, such as egg yolk. Recently, the RDA of folic acid was raised from 200 to 400 µg. Folic acid fortification of grain products has increased the percentage of the US population with adequate folate intakes (Jacques et al. 1999), but a substantial portion of the US population still has a suboptimal intake of folic acid, especially women of child-bearing age (Bajorunas 1999). Increasing evidence suggests that folate may have the potential to prevent CVD, because folic acid and other B vitamins are the primary determinants of plasma concentrations of homocysteine (Boushey et al. 1995).

Several epidemiological studies examined the association between folate intake and risk of CVD. A case-control study of 130 myocardial infarction patients and 118 control subjects by Verhoef et al. (1996) found that folate intake was significantly lower in patients than in controls. The odds ratio (OR) comparing extreme quintiles (> 682 compared with 310 µg/day) of total folate intake (supplement plus food) was 0.38 (95% CI, 0.15–0.95). The OR comparing extreme quintiles (> 467 compared with 282 µg/day) of folate from food only was 0.30 (95% CI, 0.11–0.81). The Nurses' Health Study (Rimm et al. 1998), which included 80 082 women who were followed up for 14 years, found a RR of CVD of 0.69 (95% CI, 0.55–0.87) for women in the highest quintile of folate intake (median, 696 μg/day) compared with those in the lowest quintile (median, 158 μg/day). Chee and Stamler (1999) reported a significant inverse association between folate intake and mortality from all causes and CVD in 6426 men from the Multiple Risk Factor Intervention Trial (MRFIT) usual care group.

Although numerous experimental studies have shown the homocysteine-lowering effects of folic acid supplementation (Boushey et al. 1995; Homocysteine Lowering Trialists' Collaboration 1998), few clinical trial data are currently available regarding the effect of folate on CVD outcomes. In a randomised, placebo-controlled trial, Vermeulen et al. (2000a) investigated the effect of folate on sub-clinical CVD in 158 healthy siblings of patients with existing CVD who received either 5 mg folic acid and 250 mg vitamin B6 or placebo for 2 years and reported that folic acid and vitamin B6 treatment resulted in a decrease in fasting homocysteine concentrations and a decreased rate of sub-clinical heart disease as assessed by abnormal exercise electro-cardiography tests (OR, 0.40; 95% CI, 0.17–0.93). In two uncontrolled studies, supplementation with folic acid and vitamin B6 reduced the risk of CVD events (coronary, peripheral or cerebral) in hyperhomocysteinaemic patients with existing CVD to the level of normohomocysteinaemic patients with existing CVD (DeJong et al. 1999; Vermeulen et al. 2000b).

Several large, on-going clinical trials using CVD end-points (myocardial infarction and stroke), such as the Norwegian study of homocysteine lowering with B vitamins in myocardial infarction (NORVIT) and the Women's Anti-oxidants and Cardiovascular Disease Study (WACS) will help to further clarify the beneficial role of folic acid in reducing clinical cardiovascular events.

7.10   B vitamins as a therapy for lowering homocysteine

One of the causes of hyperhomocysteinaemia is an inadequate intake of folate and the vitamins B12 and B6. Figure 7.1 shows the essential role played by these dietary micronutrients as cofactors in the metabolism of homocysteine to methionine and cysteine.

Woodside et al. (1998) carried out a double-blind, randomised, factorial design, controlled trial, in which they supplemented 101 men every day for 8 weeks with B-group vitamins (1 mg folate, 7.2 mg vitamin B6, 0.02 mg vitamin B12), antioxidant vitamins alone (150 mg ascorbate, 67 mg α-tocopherol, 9 mg β-carotene), or both. They found that supplementation with the B-group vitamins with or without antioxidants significantly ($P < 0.001$) reduced (by 27.9%) homocysteine in the men with mildly elevated total homocysteine concentration, but there was no evidence of an interaction with antioxidant vitamins combined.

The efficacy of B-group vitamins in lowering homocysteine levels was corroborated by the results of a meta-analysis carried out by the Homocysteine Lowering Trialists' Collaboration (1998). It was found that folate had the dominant blood homocysteine lowering effect, and this effect was greater among subjects with higher blood total homocysteine concentrations or lower blood folate concentrations before treatment. The authors concluded that in typical Western populations, daily supplementation with both 0.5–5 mg folic acid and about 0.5 mg vitamin B12 would be expected to reduce blood homocysteine concentrations by about one-quarter to one-third (i.e. from about 12 μmol/l to 8–9 μmol/l).

7.11 Hyperhomocysteinaemia and cardiovascular disease: cause or effect?

It may be said that hyperhomocysteinaemia is strongly associated with risk for atherothrombotic disease. However, the real question remains as to whether raised homocysteine is a causal factor or merely a secondary marker of risk. Several plausible biological mechanisms exist to explain a contribution of hyperhomocysteinaemia to atherothrombotic disease risk. These involve effects upon platelets, the coagulation system, endothelium (Bellamy et al. 1998a; Chambers et al. 1999b) and the blood vessel wall (Ueland et al. 2000). The most established theory is that of the inhibitory effect of homocysteine on nitric oxide-mediated vasodilatation. Impaired endothelial vasodilatation is well known as a precursor to vascular damage and atherosclerosis. However, most studies demonstrating this effect have been done *in vitro* or in volunteers using homocysteine concentrations at least ten times greater than those seen in patients with moderate hyperhomocysteinaemia, and should therefore be interpreted with caution (Hankey & Eikelboom 1999). Hyperhomocysteinaemia has also been suggested to play a role in the release of reactive oxygen species resulting in oxidative damage to arterial endothelial cells (Hankey & Eikelboom 1999; Brattstrom & Wilcken 2000; El Kossi & Mahrous 2000).

Theories for a role of hyperhomocysteinaemia in vascular damage are equally opposed by theories suggesting the opposite, that raised plasma homocysteine is usually benign and is a consequence rather than a cause of atherosclerosis (Brattstrom & Wilcken 2000). Plasma homocysteine concentrations are also known to be elevated in patients with impaired renal function (Brattstrom et al. 1992; Brattstrom & Wilcken 2000) due to reduced clearance in the urine via the trans-sulphuration pathway. Atherosclerosis may also cause kidney dysfunction due to nephrosclerosis, thereby increasing plasma homocysteine concentration as a consequence of the disease.

There are many ongoing prospective, controlled intervention trials using folate, vitamin B12 and vitamin B6 as homocysteine-lowering agents (Brattstrom & Wilcken 2000), the results of which may provide important information as to whether these vitamins can protect against vascular diseases. However, even if homocysteine-lowering therapies prove effective, the question of whether the beneficial effect can be ascribed to a reduction in homocysteine or to an independent effect of the B-vitamins themselves remains unresolved.

7.12 Summary

For many years now, moderately raised concentrations of total homocysteine have been associated with an increased risk of atherothrombotic vascular events. Atherothrombotic vascular diseases are a common cause of stroke, as well as of coronary heart disease. It is only recently that sufficient evidence has accumulated to suggest that the association of hyperhomocysteinaemia with vascular disease is independent and dose-related, but it remains to be established whether it is causal and modifiable. There are also some observations which suggest that mild homocysteinaemia could be an effect rather than a cause of atherosclerotic disease. There are many ongoing prospective, controlled intervention trials using folate, vitamin B12 and vitamin B6 as homocysteine-lowering agents, the results of which may provide important information as to whether these vitamins can be protective against cardiovascular diseases including stroke.

8 Endothelial Dysfunction in Stroke Disease: Potential Role of Dietary Factors

8.1 Introduction

Available evidence suggests that cardiovascular diseases, including acute ischaemic stroke, may involve endothelial dysfunction. The main functions of the vascular endothelium are to maintain blood circulation and fluidity, regulate vascular tone, and modulate leukocyte and platelet adhesion and leukocyte transmigration (Brown & Hu 2001). The endothelium is essential to the haemostatic processes of cell adhesion and migration, thrombosis and fibrinolysis. Endothelial cells express adhesion molecules, such as P-selectin, E-selectin, intercellular adhesion molecule 1 (ICAM-1) and vascular cell adhesion molecule 1 (VCAM-1), on the cell surface; these are involved in leukocyte recruitment and platelet adhesion during thrombosis and inflammation (Springer 1994). In addition, endothelial cells synthesise plasma proteins, such as von Willebrand factor (vWF), for platelet adhesion in thrombosis, and soluble molecules such as E-selectin and thrombomodulin (Vane et al. 1995). Endothelial activation can be triggered by a variety of inflammatory stimuli encountered in the blood, including oxidised low density lipoprotein (LDL), free radical species, lipopolysaccharides, and cytokines such as tumour necrosis factor. Under normal physiological conditions, endothelial activation is transient and its duration depends on the presence of the inflammatory stimulus. The activated endothelium plays an integral role in the development of atherosclerosis (Ross 1999).

The endothelial monolayer is also important for smooth muscle cell function, vascular remodelling, and the maintenance of vascular tone and vasodilatation (Cooke 2000). The endothelium synthesises several molecules that are crucial for its vasomotor function and that can be released in response to local mechanical stimuli, metabolic conditions such as hypoxia, and receptor-mediated agonists such as acetylcholine (Vogel 1997). The major endothelial products that function as vasoconstrictors are thromboxane A2, prostaglandin H2 and endothelin-1 (ET-1) (Shimokawa 1999). The endothelium-derived vasodilators include nitric oxide, endothelium-derived hyperpolarising factor and prostacyclin. Vascular tone is determined by the balance between vasoconstriction and vasodilatation agents in the environment surrounding the endothelium (Cooke 2000). Nitric oxide or endothelium-derived relaxing factor, a molecule synthesised from L-arginine by nitric oxide synthase, is the primary compound responsible for vasodilatation in arteries (Moncada & Higgs 1993). Nitric oxide inhibits platelet aggregation (Moncada & Higgs 1993), modulates leukocyte-endothelium interactions by altering cell adhesion molecule expression and reducing monocyte adherence (Tsao et al. 1996), and inhibits the proliferation of smooth muscle cells.

8.2 Endothelial dysfunction in cardiovascular disease including stroke

The two primary clinical measurements of endothelial dysfunction are enhanced and maintained endothelial activation, and impaired endothelium-dependent vasodilatation (Brown & Hu 2001). Endothelial activation is detected by increased plasma concentrations of soluble adhesion molecules such as ICAM-1, VCAM-1, and E- and P-selectin, which are shed and released into plasma from the activated endothelium and macrophages. Higher concentrations of these soluble molecules have been found in patients with diabetes and hyperlipidaemia and in persons with inflammatory conditions (Meydani, 2000; Brown & Hu 2001).

Many studies have shown that plasma concentrations of soluble cell adhesion molecules are elevated in patients with cardiovascular disease (CVD). Hwang et al. (1997) reported significantly higher circulating ICAM-1 in patients with coronary heart disease (CHD) or carotid artery atherosclerosis than in control subjects. Morisaki et al. (1997) also found elevated serum concentrations of ICAM-1 in patients with ischaemic heart disease. In addition, Peter et al. (1997) found that VCAM-1 concentrations correlated well with the extent of atherosclerosis. Ridker et al. (1998) reported that higher serum concentrations of ICAM-1 predicted future risk of myocardial infarction in the Physicians' Health Study. Several studies also showed elevated concentrations of E-selectin, VCAM-1 and ICAM-1 in subjects with diabetes (Albertini et al. 1998; Bannan et al. 1998; Ceriello et al. 1998).

Major CVD risk factors, such as smoking, hypercholesterolaemia, hypertension, diabetes and hyperhomocysteinaemia, have all been found to cause endothelial dysfunction. Smoking reduces nitric oxide production and possibly increases nitric oxide degradation as a result of increased oxidative stress (Higman et al. 1996). In addition, smokers tend to have higher concentrations of ICAM-1 and P-selectin than do non-smokers (Blann et al. 1997; Bergmann et al. 1998). Hypercholesterolaemia decreases nitric oxide production in human endothelial cells *in vitro* (Feron et al. 1999). Oxidised LDL leads to an increased expression of adhesion molecules on the endothelial cell surface, allowing for and potentiating monocyte infiltration to the sub-endothelium (Ross 1999). Conversely, high density lipoprotein (HDL) provides an atheroprotective effect by inhibiting cytokine-induced endothelial cell adhesion molecule expression (Cockerill et al. 1995) and by enhancing agonist-induced vasodilatation in coronary arteries (Kuhn et al. 1991). Diabetes mellitus is associated with physiological changes that potentiate endothelial dysfunction, such as hypertriglyceridaemia, small LDL size, low HDL, hypertension and hyperglycaemia (Verges 1999).

8.3 Endothelial dysfunction in ischaemic stroke

Animal models of cerebral ischaemia and some human studies indicate that inflammatory mechanisms contribute to secondary neuronal injury after acute cerebral ischaemia. Ischaemia followed by reperfusion leads to the expression of inflammatory cytokines, such as tumour necrosis factor and interleukin-1, which stimulate a complex cascade of events involving local endothelial, other neuronal and perivascular cells. A secondary response includes the release of other cytokines, an increase in the components of the coagulation system, an upregulation of cell adhesion molecule expression and changes in the expression of the immune system. The net effect of these events is transformation of the local endothelium to a prothrombotic/proinflammatory state and induction of leucocyte migration to the site of injury (DeGraba 1998).

Experimental studies of cerebral ischaemia and reperfusion injury demonstrate early expression of adhesion molecules (DeGraba 1998). For example, Clark et al. (1995), showed that the expression of ICAM-1 was significantly elevated on the microvasculature within 1 hour after global ischaemia in rats and that this persisted for several days. Okada et al. (1994) demonstrated that cerebral ischaemia followed by reperfusion in a primate model induced an increase in P-selectin and ICAM-1 expression on post-capillary microvessels within 1–4 hours of focal ischaemia. In addition, in a human autopsy study in which death occurred within 15 hours to 18 days after an acute stroke, Lindsberg et al. (1996) found that granulocyte density was 11.3 cells/mm^2 in the infarcted region versus 0.5 cells/mm^2 in the control area as early as 15 hours after ischaemia, and exceeded 200 cells/mm^2 by 2.2 days. Up to 97% of the microvessels stained positively for ICAM-1 by 1.8 days, demonstrating a correlation between significant ICAM-1 upregulation and leukocyte migration.

Markers of endothelial dysfunction such as ET-1 (Lampl et al. 1997), vWF (Lip et al. 2001), ICAM, VCAM (Fassbender et al. 1995) and selectins (Frijins et al. 1997) have all been shown to be increased in the plasma following acute ischaemic stroke. These are substances that are produced within the endothelium and may have various deleterious effects such as vasoconstriction, and platelet and leucocyte aggregation, which may exacerbate the ischaemic injury, but may be partly reversible (DeGraba, 1998).

Lampl et al. (1997) studied 26 patients with acute stroke, each of whom underwent two repeat computed tomography (CT) scans. Within 5–18 hours of stroke onset, lumbar puncture and blood samples were concomitantly obtained and tested for ET-1. ET-1 levels in cerebrospinal fluid (CSF) and plasma of these patients were analysed by radioimmunoassay and compared with the levels of a control group of patients with no neurological disease; ET-1 was significantly elevated in the CSF of stroke patients during 18 hours after stroke, with no elevation being demonstrated in plasma during this period. Lampl et al. (1997) hypothesised that the dissimilarity between CSF and plasma ET-1 may be due to a vasoconstrictive effect on the cerebral vessels or a neuronal effect caused by ET-1 in the mechanism of progression of brain ischaemia.

Lip et al. (2001) investigated abnormalities of haemorrheology (plasma viscosity, fibrinogen), endothelial dysfunction (vWF), platelet activation (soluble P-selectin) and thrombogenesis (plasminogen activator inhibitor and fibrin D-dimer) in 86 patients younger than 75 years within 12 hours of acute stroke. Baseline blood tests on admission were compared with 46 'hospital controls' who were patients with uncomplicated essential hypertension aged 65.9 ± 3.8 years, and 24 healthy normotensive controls aged 65 ± 14.0 years. Further comparisons were made between stroke patients with hypertension (systolic blood pressure above 160 mmHg and/or diastolic pressure above 90 mmHg) on admission and those without hypertension. Their study revealed clear abnormalities of haemorrheology, endothelial dysfunction, platelet activation and thrombogenesis, which did not appear to be affected by the height of the blood pressure or the presence of hypertension.

An increase in concentrations of serum ICAM-1 and decreased levels of serum L-selectin were also found in patients with risk factors, even in the absence of stroke. Patients with acute stroke had, in addition, an initial transient increase of serum ICAM-1 and a persistent increase of VCAM-1 (Fassbender et al. 1995).

In another study of 28 acute ischaemic stroke patients, 34 patients with transient or persistent ischaemic neurological deficit associated with stenosis of the internal carotid artery and 34 control patients without a history of vascular disease, Frijns et al. (1997) reported that, compared with control subjects, P-selectin and serum E-selectin were significantly elevated in the acute stage of the stroke and in patients with symptomatic carotid stenosis; ICAM-1 and serum VCAM-1 were not increased.

De Graba et al. (1998) have studied ICAM-1 expression in carotid plaques from 25 symptomatic and 17 asymptomatic patients undergoing carotid endarterectomy; an elevation in ICAM-1 expression in symptomatic versus asymptomatic plaque suggested that mediators of inflammation are involved in the conversion of carotid plaque to a symptomatic state. The data also suggested differential expression of ICAM-1, with greater expression being found in the high-grade region than in the low-grade region of the plaque specimen.

Endothelium dysfunction may therefore have various deleterious effects, such as vasoconstriction, and platelet and leucocyte aggregation, which may exacerbate ischaemic injury following stroke, but may also be partly reversible through dietary means.

8.4   Dietary factors influencing endothelial dysfunction

Recently there has been growing interest in the role of dietary and nutritional factors, such as n-3 fatty acids (which include omega-3 fatty acids), antioxidant vitamins, folic acid and L-arginine, in modulating endothelial function.

8.4.1   Effects of antioxidant vitamin supplementation on endothelial function

In CVD, antioxidants reduce the susceptibility of LDL to oxidation and scavenge free radicals within the body, reducing the overall oxidative status of a person (Pryor 2000). Emerging evidence has also suggested a possible role for antioxidants in modulating endothelial function, which is probably partly mediated by their antioxidant activity. In animal models, α-tocopherol was found to preserve nitric oxide-mediated vascular relaxation (Anderson et al. 1994; Stewart-Lee et al. 1994). *In vitro* studies showed a reduction in cell adhesion molecule expression (Wu et al. 1999), monocyte adhesion to the endothelium (Faruqi et al. 1994) and improvement in endothelium-dependent vasodilatation (Fontana et al. 1999) after incubation of endothelial cells with antioxidants.

In addition to the *in vitro* evidence, there is growing clinical evidence to support a favourable effect of antioxidants on endothelial function (Aminbakhsh & Mancini 1999). Table 8.1 shows studies of the effects of antioxidant supplementation on endothelial function, ranging in duration from 1 week to 3 months and using either vitamin C or vitamin E supplementation. High doses of vitamins E and C decreased soluble markers of endothelial activation, such as P-selectin, and reduced monocyte adhesion (Devaraj et al. 1996; Weber et al. 1996; Davi et al. 1998; Seljeflot et al. 1998).

Single-dose parenteral administration of antioxidant vitamins reduced endothelial dysfunction in different patient populations, including chronic smokers (Heitzer et al. 1996), patients with diabetes (Ting et al. 1997), with hypertension (Ting et al. 1997) and with chronic heart failure (Hornig et al. 1998). Several studies have assessed the relatively long-term effect of antioxidant oral supplementation on endothelium-dependent vasodilatation.

Table 8.1 Clinical studies of antioxidant vitamins and endothelial function. Reproduced from Brown & Hu (2001) with permission from *American Journal of Clinical Nutrition*. © American Society for Clinical Nutrition.

Reference	Year	Study design[a]	Subjects	Antioxidant and daily dosage	Duration	Methods[b]	Outcome
Endothelial adhesive properties							
Devaraj et al.	1996	p	Healthy subjects (*n* = 21)	1200 IU tocopherol	8 weeks	Monocyte adhesion assay	Decreased monocyte adhesion
Weber et al.	1996	p	Smokers (*n* = 10), non-smokers (*n* = 6)	2000 mg vitamin C	10 days	Monocyte adhesion assay	Decreased monocyte adhesion
Seljeflot et al.	1998	p, r, p-c	Smokers with hyperlipidaemia (*n* = 41)	150 mg vitamin C, 75 mg vitamin E and 15 mg β-carotene	6 weeks	Plasma TM, vWF, P-selectin, E-selectin, VCAM-1	No improvement
Davi et al.	1998	p	Subjects with hypercholesterolaemia (*n* = 20)	600 mg 2-epi-l-tocopherol	2 weeks	Plasma P-selectin	Reduction in P-selectin
Endothelial-dependent vasodilatation							
Hornig et al.	1998	p, p-c	Subjects with chronic heart failure (*n* = 10)	2 g vitamin C or placebo	4 weeks	Flow-mediated dilatation of radial artery	Improvement
Motoyama et al.	1998	p, r, p-c	Subjects with coronary spastic angina (*n* = 60)	300 mg tocopherol plus 200 mg diltiazem or diltiazem plus placebo	4 weeks	Flow-mediated dilatation of brachial artery	Improvement

Author	Year	Design[a]	Subjects	Dose	Duration	Method	Outcome
Kugiyama et al.	1999	p, r, p-c	Patients with high remnant lipoprotein (n = 70)	300 IU tocopherol	4 weeks	Flow-mediated dilatation of brachial artery	Improvement
Gocke et al.	1999	p, r, p-c	CAD patients (n = 46)	500 mg vitamin C	4 weeks	Flow-mediated dilatation of brachial artery	Improvement
Chambers et al.	1999	p, r, p-c	Healthy subjects (n = 17)	1000 mg vitamin C	1 week	Flow-mediated dilatation of brachial artery	Improvement
Simons et al.	1999	p, r, p-c	Healthy subjects (n = 20)	1000 IU vitamin E	10 weeks	Flow-mediated dilatation of brachial artery	No improvement
Raitakari et al.	2000	p, r, p-c	Smokers (n = 20)	1000 mg vitamin C	8 weeks	Flow-mediated dilatation of brachial artery	No improvement
Neunteufl et al.	2000	p, r, p-c	Smokers (n = 22)	600 IU vitamin E	4 weeks	Flow-mediated dilatation of brachial artery	Improvement
Skyrme-Jones et al.	2000	p, r, p-c	Patients with type 1 diabetes (n = 41)	1000 IU vitamin E	3 months	Flow-mediated dilatation of brachial artery	Improvement

[a] p, prospective; r, randomised; p-c, placebo-controlled.
[b] TM, thrombomodulin; ICAM-I, intercellular adhesion molecule 1; VCAM-1, vascular cell adhesion module 1; CAD coronary artery disease; vWF von Willebrand factor.

Hornig et al. (1998) found that flow-mediated vasodilatation was significantly improved after 4 weeks of oral supplementation with vitamin C (2 g/day) in patients with heart failure, which was partly mediated by increased availability of nitric oxide; however, flow-mediated vasodilatation was not affected by vitamin C in healthy control subjects. The benefit of vitamin C supplementation on endothelium-mediated vasodilatation was also shown in patients with existing CHD by Gocke et al. (1999). A study by Chambers et al. (1999a) revealed that pre-treatment with vitamin C (1 g/day orally for 1 week) was effective in ameliorating a reduction in flow-mediated vasodilatation induced by acute hyperhomocysteinaemia in healthy subjects. In contrast with these studies showing relatively long-term effects of vitamin C, Raitakari et al. (2000) found that although a single dose of vitamin C improved vascular function in the short term in adult smokers with baseline endothelial dysfunction, vitamin C supplementation (1 g/day) for 8 weeks had no significant benefit, despite sustained elevated concentrations of plasma vitamin C. Vitamin E supplementation was also shown to improve endothelium-dependent vasodilatation in several studies. Motoyama et al. (1998) found that vitamin E treatment (300 mg α-tocopherol/day) for 4 weeks improved endothelium-dependent vasodilatation and decreased plasma thiobarbituric acid reactive substance (TBARS) concentrations in 60 patients with documented coronary spastic angina. Kugiyama et al. (1999) found that treatment with α-tocopherol (300 IU/day) for 4 weeks significantly improved impaired endothelium-dependent vasodilatation in patients with high remnant concentrations, the improvement being associated with decreased plasma concentrations of TBARS. This finding suggests that the beneficial effects of vitamin E on endothelial dysfunction were partly mediated by a reduction in oxidative stress with vitamin E therapy. Neunteufl et al. (2000) found that vitamin E supplementation (600 IU/day) for 4 weeks did not restore endothelial dysfunction caused by smoking in 22 healthy male smokers. However, pretreatment with vitamin E was effective in preventing a further decline in endothelium-dependent vasodilatation in the brachial artery induced by acute smoking. Only two studies lasted 10 weeks or more: Simons et al. (1999) found that supplementation with vitamin E (1000 IU/day) for 10 weeks did not affect flow-mediated endothelium-dependent dilation in response to reactive hyperaemia in 20 asymptomatic subjects aged 45–70 years, whereas Skyrme-Jones et al. (2000) showed in a study lasting 3 months that 1000 IU/day of vitamin E significantly improved flow-mediated vasodilatation in the brachial artery and flow responses to intrabrachial acetylcholine in the forearm resistance vessels in subjects with type 1 diabetes. Taken together, the results of most of the studies support a role for vitamins C and E in preserving endothelium-dependent vasodilatation when challenged with cardiovascular risk factors such as hyperlipidaemia or in patients with diabetes or established CVD. In several of the studies, the improvement in endothelial function was directly related to a reduction in oxidative stress, supporting the theory that the benefit of these vitamins on endothelial function is at least partly mediated by their antioxidant property.

8.4.2   Effects of folic acid on endothelial function

The primary mechanism proposed for the effect of folic acid on CVD is a reduction in plasma homocysteine concentrations by remethylation of homocysteine back to methionine (Haynes 1999). There is increasing evidence that folic acid can have a beneficial effect on the vascular endothelium by reducing plasma homocysteine concentrations or through other mechanisms such as reduction of oxidative stress (Wilmink et al. 2000).

As discussed in Chapter 7, homocysteine harms the vascular endothelium in a variety of ways, impairing its ability to maintain homeostasis. Homocysteine increases platelet aggregation and thrombosis through enhanced thromboxane synthesis and inactivation of anticoagulant substances (Haynes 1999); it increases oxidative stress by elevating superoxide production (McDowell & Lang 2000) and also enhances leukocyte–endothelium interactions; it was found to be toxic at high concentrations (Dudman et al. 1999). In addition, homocysteine downregulates nitric oxide production (Pruefer et al. 1999) and acts as a mitogen to increase vascular smooth muscle proliferation (Tsai et al. 1994).

Impaired endothelium-dependent, flow-mediated vasodilatation was documented in hyperhomocysteinaemic subjects (Tawakol et al. 1997; Woo et al. 1997), and in healthy subjects with oral methionine load-induced hyper-homocysteinaemia (Bellamy et al. 1998; Chambers et al. 1999a, b).

Acute administration of folic acid can restore impaired endothelial function induced by acute hyperhomocysteinaemia (Usui et al. 1999). Table 8.2 shows several relatively long-term studies (2–12 weeks) evaluating the effects of folic acid supplementation on endothelial function. In a study of 18 mildly hyper-homocysteinaemic patients with peripheral arterial occlusive disease, Van den Berg et al. (1995) found that daily treatment with pyridoxine (250 mg) plus folic acid (5 mg) significantly decreased concentrations of vWF and throm-bomodulin after 12 weeks of treatment. Woo et al. (1999) found that supple-mentation with 10 mg/day folic acid for 8 weeks significantly improved flow-mediated endothelium-dependent vasodilatation in 17 healthy subjects with relative hyperhomocystinaemia (mean homocysteine concentration 9.8 mmol/l). Verhaar et al. (1999) assessed supplementation with 5 mg folic acid for 4 weeks on serotonin-induced blood flow in patients with familial hypercho-lesterolaemia and found that it restored endothelium-dependent vasodilata-tion in these patients to normal control levels. Bellamy et al. (1999) noted a significant improvement in endothelium-dependent vasodilatation in hyper-

Table 8.2 Clinical studies of folic acid supplementation and endothelial function. Reproduced from Brown & Hu (2001) with permission from *American Journal of Clinical Nutrition*. American Society for Clinical Nutrition.

Reference	Year	Study design	Subjects	Daily dosage	Duration	Methods[b]	Outcome[b]
Van den Berg et al.	1995	p	Mildly hyperhomocysteinaemic subjects (n=18)	(5 mg) folic acid + (250 mg) pyridoxine	12 weeks	Measurement of plasma vWF, TM	Decreased vWF, TM
Woo et al.	1999	p, r, p-c	Healthy subjects (n=17)	10 mg folic acid or placebo	8 weeks	Measurement of flow-mediated vasodilatation of brachial artery	Improved endothelium-dependent vasodilatation
Verhaar et al	1999	p, r, p-c	Familial hypercholesterolaemic (n=40)	5 mg folic acid or placebo	4 weeks	Serotonin-induced forearm blood flow measurement	Restored endothelium-dependent vasodilatation
Bellamy et al.	1999	p, r, p-c	Hyperhomocysteinaemic patients (n=18)	5 mg folic acid or placebo	6 weeks	Measurement of flow-mediated vasodilatation of brachial artery	Improved endothelium-dependent vasodilitation
Constans et al.	1999	p	Hyperhomocysteinaemic patients and control subjects (n=44)	5 mg folic acid and 250 mg vitamin B6	3 months	Plasma TM, vWF measurement	Decreased TM
Wilmink et al.	2000	p, r, p-c	Healthy subjects postprandially (n=20)	10 mg folic acid or placebo	2 weeks	Measurement of flow-mediated vasodilatation of brachial artery	Prevention of vasodilatation impairment after fat load
Thambyrajah et al.	2000	p, r, p-c	Patients with pre-dialysis renal failure (n=100)	5 mg folic acid or placebo	12 weeks	Measurement of flow-mediated vasodilatation of brachial artery vWF	No change

[a] p, prospective; r, randomised; p-c, placebo-controlled.
[b] TM, thrombomodulin; vWF, von Willebrand factor

homocysteinaemic patients after supplementation with 5 mg/day folic acid for 6 weeks. Constans et al. (1999) found a significant reduction in thrombo-modulin after supplementation with folic acid (5 mg/day) and vitamin B6 (250 mg/day) for 3 months of hyperhomocysteinaemic patients. Wilmink et al. (2000) evaluated the effect of pretreatment with 10 mg/day folic acid or placebo for 2 weeks on postprandial endothelial dysfunction after an oral fat load. The oral fat load resulted in an increase in triacylglycerol concentrations in both treated and placebo groups, and impaired flow-mediated vasodilata-tion in the placebo group but not the supplemented group. Urinary mal-ondialdehyde, a measure of oxidative stress, was significantly elevated in the placebo group but not in the folic acid-treated group. Thambyrajah et al. (2000) evaluated the effects of supplementation with 5 mg/day folic acid or placebo for 12 weeks on endothelial dysfunction in 100 patients with pre-dialysis renal failure. Endothelial dysfunction was assessed by measuring:

(1)   Endothelium-dependent dilation of the brachial artery.
(2)   Combined serum nitrite and nitrate concentrations.
(3)   Plasma vWF concentrations.

The treatment lowered but did not normalise hyperhomocysteinaemia in these patients, and there was no significant change in any of the three measures of endothelial dysfunction. The authors concluded that treatment with high doses of folic acid might not be able to reverse endothelial dysfunction in patients with renal failure.

The overall results of these studies suggest that folic acid supplementation has a beneficial effect on endothelial function, as measured by flow-mediated vasodilatation or homeostatic markers, in healthy subjects or patients with elevated homocysteine. The observed benefit is probably explained largely by the homocysteine-lowering effect of folic acid; however, other mechanisms may contribute to the benefit. A previous study showed that acute adminis-tration of folic acid improved endothelial function without any effects on homocysteine concentrations (Verhaar et al. 1998). Folic acid was shown to have antioxidant properties and direct scavenging effects *in vitro* (Verhaar et al. 1998), and may directly improve nitric oxide production by enhancing enzymatic activity of nitric oxide synthase (Stroes et al. 2000).

8.4.3   Effects of n-3 fatty acids on endothelial function

The exact mechanism by which n-3 fatty acids exert an atheroprotective effect is unclear. However, n-3 fatty acids can influence many aspects of the pathogenesis of CVD, including lipid concentrations, the size and oxidisability of lipids (Harris 1989), platelet aggregation (von Shacky 2000) and arrhythmia (Kang & Leaf 2000). There is growing evidence regarding the beneficial effects of fish oil on endothelial function (De Caterina et al. 2000; Goodfellow et al. 2000).

There are several *in vitro* studies that have examined the effects of n-3 fatty acids on cell adhesion molecule surface and mRNA expression, as well as leukocyte and endothelium interactions (De Caterina et al. 1994, 1998; Weber et al. 1995; Khalfoun et al. 1996). Overall, these studies showed that n-3 fatty acids decrease expression of VCAM-1 on the vascular endothelium and decrease leukocyte rolling and adhesion to the endothelium. Although the results of these *in vitro* studies are consistent in supporting a favourable effect of n-3 fatty acids on endothelial function, results from *in vivo* studies are less consistent.

Table 8.3 shows five *in vivo* studies examining n-3 supplementation and measures of endothelial function, the results of which contradict the results of the *in vitro* studies listed above which clearly showed that n-3 fatty acids reduce expression of cytokine-induced adhesion molecules. There is also some evidence that highly concentrated n-3 fatty acids in fish oil may be prone to peroxidation (Frankel et al. 1994), which can stimulate expression of endothelial cell adhesion molecules. Thus, Johansen et al. (1999) suggested that a high dose of fish oil without adequate protection by antioxidant vitamins might induce proinflammatory responses and adversely affect endothelial function.

Two studies have examined the effects of n-3 fatty acid supplementation on endothelium-dependent vasomotor function. Fleischhauer et al. (1993) assessed the effects of dietary supplementation of n-3 fatty acid on endothelium-dependent vasodilator responses of coronary arteries to intracoronary acetylcholine infusion in heart transplant recipients. After 3 weeks of treatment, patients treated with fish oil improved their vasodilator response to normal levels, whereas control patients showed vasoconstrictor response. Goodfellow et al. (2000) randomly assigned 30 hypercholesterolaemic subjects either to a group treated with 4 g/day n-3 fatty acids or to a placebo group. At baseline, the hypercholesterolaemic patients exhibited impaired endothelium-dependent vasodilatation compared with the healthy subjects, but after 4 months of treatment, the patients supplemented with n-3 fatty acids had significantly improved endothelium-dependent vasodilatation compared with the control subjects. The mechanisms by which n-3 fatty acids influence the function of endothelium are still under investigation.

8.4.4 ʟ-Arginine and endothelial function

ʟ-Arginine is a semiessential amino acid that is important during periods of growth and is required for the urea cycle in protein catabolism (Niittynen et al. 1999). ʟ-Arginine is also the substrate for nitric oxide synthase in the

Table 8.3 Clinical studies of n-3 fatty acids and endothelial function. Reproduced from Brown & Hu (2001) with permission from *American Journal of Clinical Nutrition*. © American Society for Clinical Nutrition.

Reference	Year	Study design[a]	Subjects	Daily dosage	Duration	Methods[b]	Outcome[b]
Fleischhauer et al.	1993	p, r, p-c	Heart transplant patients ($n = 14$)	5 g omega-3 fatty acids	3 weeks	ACH-mediated dilatation of coronary arteries	Improved vasodilatation
Abe et al.	1998	p, r, p-c	Hypertriglyceridaemic subjects ($n = 39$)	4 g omega-3 fatty acids (Omacor)	6 weeks, 7 months	ICAM-1, VCAM-1, E-selectin	Decreased ICAM-1 and E-selectin after 7 months
Seljeflot et al.	1998	p, r, p-c	Smokers with hyperlipidaemia ($n = 41$)	4.8 g omega-3 fatty acids	6 weeks	TM, vWF, P-selectin, E-selectin, VCAM-1	Decreased TM and vWF; increased VCAM-1 and E-selectin
Johansen et al.	1999	p, r	CHD patients ($n = 54$)	5.1 g omega-3 fatty acids	4 weeks	TM, vWF, P-selectin, E-selectin, VCAM-1	Decreased TM and vWF; increased VCAM-1 and E-selectin
Goodfellow et al.	2000	p, r, p-c	Hypercholesterolaemic subjects ($n = 30$)	4 g omega-3 fatty acids	120 days	Flow-mediated dilatation of brachial artery	Improved vasodilatation

[a] p, prospective; r, randomised; p-c; placebo-controlled.
[b] ACH, aceytlcholine; ICAM-1, intercellular adhesion molecule 1; VCAM-1, vascular cell adhesion molecule 1; TM, soluble thrombomodulin; vWF, von Willebrand factor.

Table 8.4 Clinical studies of L-arginine supplementation and endothelial function. Reproduced from Brown & Hu (2001) from *American Journal of Clinical Nutrition*. © American Society for Clinical Nutrition.

Reference	Year	Study design[a]	Subjects[b]	Daily dosage	Duration	Methods[c]	Outcome
Adams et al.	1997	p, r, p-c	CHD patients ($n = 10$)	21 g L-arginine or placebo	3 days	Flow-mediated dilatation of brachial artery	Improvement
						Monocyte adhesion assay	Reduced monocyte–endothelium adhesion
Clarkson et al.	1996	p, r, p-c	Hypercholesterolaemic patients ($n = 27$)	21 g L-arginine or placebo	4 weeks	Flow-mediated dilatation of brachial artery	Improvement
Theilmeier et al	1997	p, r, p-c	Hypercholesterolaemic patients and control subjects ($n = 32$)	8.4 g arginine HCl	2 weeks	Monocyte adhesion assay	Reduced monocyte–endothelium adhesion
Bellamy et al.	1998b	p, r, p-c	Angina patients and control subjects ($n = 17$)	14 g L-arginine or placebo	4 weeks	Flow-mediated dilatation of brachial artery	Improvement
Lerman et al.	1998	p, r, p-c	Recurrent chest pain patients ($n = 26$)	9 g L-arginine or placebo	6 months	Agonist (ACH)-mediated coronary blood flow	Improvement
Hambrecht et al.	2000	p, r	Chronic heart failure patients ($n = 20$)	8 g L-arginine	4 weeks	Agonist (ACH)-mediated dilatation of radial artery	Improvement

Study	Year	Design	Population	Intervention	Duration	Measure	Outcome
Mullen et al.	2000	p, r, p-c	Patients with type 1 diabetes (n = 84)	14 g L-arginine	6 weeks	Flow-mediated dilatation of brachial artery	No improvement
Blum et al.	1999	p	Patients with intractable angina pectoris (n = 10)	9 g L-arginine	3 months	Soluble ICAM-1, VCAM-1, E-, P- and L-selectin	Reduction in plasma ICAM-1, P- and E-selectin concentrations
Blum et al.	2000a	p, r, p-c	CHD patients (n = 29)	9 g L-arginine or placebo	1 month	Flow-mediated dilatation of brachial artery	No improvement
						Soluble ICAM-1, VCAM-1, E-selectin	No change
Blum et al.	2000b	p, r, p-c	Post-menopausal women (n = 10)	9 g L-arginine or placebo	1 month	Flow-mediated dilatation of brachial artery	No improvement
						Soluble ICAM-1, VCAM-1, E-selectin	No change

[a] p, prospective; r, randomised; p-c, placebo-controlled.
[b] CHD, coronary heart disease.
[c] ACH, acetylcholine; ICAM-1, intercellular adhesion molecule 1; VCAM-1, vascular cell adhesion molecule 1.

production of nitric oxide and is therefore essential for the maintenance of proper vascular function. In hypercholesterolaemic animal models, dietary supplementation with L-arginine improves endothelium-dependent dilatation, decreases platelet aggregation and monocyte adhesion, and reduces the development of atherosclerosis (Adams et al. 1997).

Table 8.4 shows several clinical experimental studies which examined the effect of L-arginine supplementation on endothelial function in humans. Clarkson et al. (1996) showed that supplementation with 21 g/day L-arginine for 4 weeks resulted in a 3.9% improvement in flow-mediated dilatation in hypercholesterolaemic patients. In coronary artery disease patients supplemented with 21 g/day L-arginine, Adams et al. (1997) found a 4.7% improvement in flow-mediated endothelium-dependent dilatation and a significant reduction in monocyte adherence to the endothelium. Theilmeier et al. (1997) supplemented hypercholesterolaemic patients and normocholesterolaemic subjects with 8.4 g/day L-arginine and assessed *ex vivo* monocyte adhesion to endothelial cells. At baseline, monocytes from the hypercholesterolaemic patients adhered by 50% more than did those from the normocholesterolaemic subjects, whereas after L-arginine supplementation, the monocytes from the hypercholesterolaemic patients had reduced adhesion comparable with control levels, suggesting that the increased adhesiveness of mononuclear cells induced by hypercholesterolaemia can be reversed *in vivo* by L-arginine. In another study, patients with angina, who had normal results of a coronary arteriogram and a positive exercise test, were supplemented with 14 g/day L-arginine for 4 weeks. These patients' flow-mediated dilatation was improved by 3.4% to physiologically normal levels (Bellamy et al. 1998b). Lerman et al. (1998) assessed coronary blood flow in patients with recurrent chest pain after supplementation with 9 g/day L-arginine or placebo for 6 months. The treatment group had a 149% greater acetylcholine-mediated coronary blood flow than the placebo group. Hambrecht et al. (2000) supplemented patients with chronic heart failure with 8 g/day L-arginine for 4 weeks and found an 8.8% improvement in acetylcholine-mediated vasodilatation of the radial artery. However, Mullen et al. (2000) found that in 84 normocholesterolaemic patients with type 1 diabetes, 7 g L-arginine twice daily had no significant effect on endothelial function as measured by flow-mediated dilatation of the brachial artery, whereas treatment with atorvastatin significantly lowered LDL cholesterol and improved endothelial dysfunction. Blum and co-workers conducted three studies in different patient populations to examine the effect of L-arginine supplementation on soluble adhesion molecule concentrations and flow-mediated dilatation. In a study of 10 patients with intractable angina pectoris (Blum et al. 1999), supplementation with 9 g/day L-arginine for 3 months resulted in a significant reduction in plasma concentrations of ICAM-1 and P- and E-selectin. However, the two other studies showed no effect of L-arginine on either flow-mediated vasodilatation or soluble adhesion molecules

(Blum et al. 2000a, b): 30 patients with coronary artery disease were randomly assigned to receive 9 g/day L-arginine or placebo for 1 month; although the plasma arginine concentration increased significantly in the treatment group, serum nitrogen oxides, flow-mediated brachial artery dilatation and concentrations of cell adhesion molecules did not change significantly (Blum et al. 2000a). In the other study, 10 healthy post-menopausal women received 9 g/day L-arginine or placebo for 1 month. The treatment had no effects on serum nitrogen oxide concentrations; flow-mediated vasodilatation and serum concentrations of soluble cell adhesion molecules were also similar between the treatment and placebo groups (Blum et al. 2000b). The authors speculated that the relatively low dosage of L-arginine used in their studies might have accounted for the lack of effect on endothelial function. Taken together, the results of these studies suggest a potential beneficial effect of L-arginine supplementation on endothelial function in patients with hypercholesterolaemia or existing coronary artery disease; however, the benefit has not been shown in subjects with diabetes or healthy subjects.

In an epidemiological study, dietary arginine intake (which is far below the supplement dosages) did not appear to predict CHD mortality (Omen et al. 2000). However, in the Nurses' Health Study (Hu et al. 1999), a moderately high consumption of dietary protein (median, 24% of energy), compared with a low consumption (median, 15% of energy), was associated with a modest but significantly lower risk of CHD during 14 years of follow-up. In several large epidemiological studies, a high consumption of nuts was associated with a significantly lower risk of CHD (Hu & Stampfer 1999). The relatively high arginine content of nuts has been suggested as one of the potential biological mechanisms for their cardioprotective effect. So far, no clinical trials have assessed the effect of supplementary arginine on cardiovascular events. Clearly, this would be an interesting and promising line of investigation.

8.5 Summary

Endothelial dysfunction, clinically assessed by measuring plasma concentrations of soluble endothelial adhesion molecules or by endothelium-dependent vasodilatation, is present in patients with all types of CVD, and also in patients who do not have clinically manifested CVD but who have risk factors such as smoking, hypertension, hypercholesterolaemia, hyperhomocysteinaemia and diabetes mellitus. Because abnormal endothelial function is an early marker of CVD, the endothelium appears to be an ideal target for preventative therapy.

Emerging and growing evidence suggests that dietary intervention is a promising strategy for improving endothelial function in patients at risk of

CVD and those with existing CVD including stroke. There is a substantial evidence to suggest that omega-3 fatty acids, antioxidant vitamins, folic acid and L-arginine have beneficial effects on endothelial function. The mechanisms by which these nutrients influence endothelial function are likely to be multiple and complex, including inhibition of monocyte adhesion and platelet activation, increased nitric oxide production, improvement of vasodilatation, and blockage of lipid oxidation. These mechanisms may contribute to the role of these nutrients in reducing the incidence of CHD that has been observed in epidemiological studies and some controlled clinical trials. The overall evidence to support the benefit of omega-3 fatty acids in CVD appears more convincing than that for other nutrients. Although definitive data on the role of antioxidants and folic acid in reducing CVD are not yet available, a balanced diet that provides a sufficient supply of these nutrients is likely to have substantial benefits for CVD, including stroke.

There is some evidence to suggest that blood vessels leading to the infarcting tissue in strokes are involved in an acute inflammatory response that promotes endothelial dysfunction. From the available evidence, acute ischaemic stroke may involve endothelial dysfunction. More clinical experimental studies are needed to elucidate the role of endothelial functions in stroke disease. Moreover, these studies need to look at the effects of dietary components on endothelial function in stroke disease.

III Nutrition Factors Following Stroke

9 Cerebral Ischaemia, Reperfusion and Oxidative Damage in Ischaemic Stroke

9.1 Introduction

The majority of strokes (about 80%) are due to cerebral infarction, 10% to primary intracerebral haemorrhage, 5% to subarachnoid haemorrhage, and in 5% the cause is uncertain (Warlow et al. 1996). There is strong indirect evidence that free radical production appears to be an important mechanism of brain injury after exposure to ischaemia and reperfusion (Wei at al. 1985; Schmidley, 1990; Traystamn et al. 1991). Body defences against free radicals depend on the balance between free radical generation and the antioxidant protective defence system. Many of these protective antioxidants are essential nutrients or have an essential nutrient that has to be obtained from diet as part of their molecule.

9.2 Cerebral ischaemia and reperfusion

Experimental models of ischaemic stroke in monkeys and cats have shown that large infarcts develop with residual flow rates of 12 ml/100 g/min lasting for 2–6 hours, and individual cells may become necrotic with lower flow values after shorter periods of time. For example, middle cerebral artery (MCA) occlusion in rats induced selective neuronal necrosis in the putamen after 15 minutes, selective neuronal necrosis in the neocortex after 30 minutes and cortical infarcts after 60 minutes. With an occlusion time of 120–180 minutes, infarct size increased and reached that found after permanent MCA occlusion (Memezawa et al. 1992; Heiss & Graf 1994). Nevertheless, animal experiments have shown that short-term recovery of electrical and metabolic function is possible with reperfusion after ischaemic periods as long as 60 minutes, and that reperfusion within 4–8 hours can reduce the size of the lesion (Jones et al. 1981; Siesjo 1992a). Using positron emission tomography (PET) scanning to differentiate between ischaemia and infarction, viable tissues in humans have been detected for up to 48 hours after the onset of stroke, but it is not yet precisely known how long ischaemic brain can survive and still be salvaged by reperfusion or other measures which protect the neurones from dying (Warlow et al. 1996).

The extent of neurological damage that occurs as a direct result of ischaemia and reperfusion depends on a number of factors. These include the amount of blood flow reduction, the duration of time that flow is reduced, the regional location of the flow reduction and the metabolic state of the brain before the ischaemic injury period (Traystamn et al. 1991).

Occlusion of a cerebral artery reduces, but seldom abolishes, the delivery of oxygen and glucose to the relevant region of the brain, because dense collateral channels partly maintain blood flow in the ischaemic territory. This incomplete ischaemia is responsible for the dynamics of cerebral infarction (Pulsinelli 1992; Warlow et al. 1996). Some other areas of the brain, including the infarcted tissues, may show relative or absolute hyperaemia (called 'luxury perfusion') due to good collateral blood supply, recanalisation of the occluded artery, inflammation or vasodilatation in response to hypercapnia, i.e. flow in excess of metabolic demands (Warlow et al. 1996). The concept of free radical damage incurred as a result of ischaemia and reperfusion (Figure 9.1) is based on the metabolic events during the ischaemia–reperfusion transition, encompassing accumulation of reduced compounds during anoxia and their oxidation when the oxygen supply is restored.

9.3   Biochemical and molecular changes following cerebral ischaemia

Using PET scanning several hours after ischaemic stroke has demonstrated an area of viable brain tissue called the ischaemic penumbra (Heiss & Graf 1994), an area of brain tissue with impaired perfusion and metabolism which is still viable and potentially salvageable by therapeutic intervention. Therefore treatment designed to improve recovery after cerebral ischaemia may be possible using biochemical and/or molecular interventions.

The mechanisms giving rise to ischaemic cell death have not been definitely determined, but there is strong evidence that three major factors are involved; these include increases in intracellular cytosolic calcium concentration (Ca^{2+}), acidosis and production of free radicals (Siesjo 1992b). Extracellular Ca^{2+} concentration is 10^4–10^5 times greater than its intracellular concentration, and most of the mechanisms that maintain this gradient are either directly or indirectly energy dependent. Therefore loss of ATP rapidly leads to a massive influx of Ca^{2+} into the cell as a result of impaired Ca^{2+} pump function (due to ATP depletion), an increase in membrane permeability to Ca^{2+}, release of Ca^{2+} from intracellular compartments, and the release of endogenous excitatory amino acid neurotransmitters (such as glutamine) from depolarised nerve endings; glutamate activates several post-synaptic glutamate receptors and/or

Some antioxidants and their actions

Vitamin E: inhibits lipid peroxidation. It appears that oxidation resistance of low density lipoprotein (LDL) as an index of susceptibility to atherosclerosis is strongly associated with its vitamin E content (Halliwell 1994).

Vitamin C: probably assists α-tocopherol in inhibition of lipid peroxidation by recycling the tocopherol radical. Good scavenger for many free radicals and also contributes to increased resistance of LDL to oxidation by recycling vitamin E (Halliwell 1994).

Superoxide dismutase (SOD): Copper/zinc dependent SOD, located in the cytoplasmic region of neurons, is the primary antioxidant involved in the conversion of the superoxide radical to hydrogen peroxide in the context of membrane damage evoked by lipid peroxidation (Cebalos-Picot et al. 1996; Pitchumoni and Doraiswamy 1998).

Catalase: converts hydrogen peroxide into water and oxygen. In the central nervous system, it is believed that free radicals such as the hydroxyl radical degrade membrane lipids through lipid peroxidation (Halliwell 1989).

Glutathione peroxidase: converts hydrogen peroxide and reduced glutathione to water and oxidised glutathione respectively (Pitchumoni and Doraiswamy 1998).

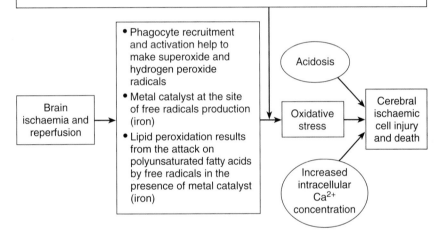

Figure 9.1   Cerebral ischaemic cell injury and oxidative stress.

channel complexes causing Na^+ influx and depolarisation, followed by more Ca^{2+} influx via ligand- and voltage-regulated ion channels (Warlow et al. 1996). A rise in Ca^{2+} resulting from a disturbed Ca^{2+} pump/leak relationship is believed to cause cell damage by overactivation of lipases and proteases (and possibly also endonucleases), and by alterations of protein phosphorylation which secondarily affects protein synthesis and genome expression. The severity of this disturbance depends on the density of ischaemia. In complete or near complete ischaemia of the cardiac arrest type, pump activity has ceased and Ca^{2+} leakage is enhanced by the massive release of excitatory amino acids. As a result, multiple calcium channels are opened. Such ischaemic tissues may only be salvaged by recirculation. If the ischaemia is less dense, however, as in the penumbral zone of a focal cerebral ischaemic lesion, pump failure may be moderate and the leak may be only slightly or intermittently enhanced. These differences in the pump/leak relationship for Ca^{2+} explain why calcium and glutamic acid antagonists may be ineffective on the cardiac arrest type of ischaemia, while decreasing the infarct size in focal ischaemia (Siesjo 1992b). Solid experimental evidence exists that the infarct resulting from MCA occlusion can be reduced by glutamic acid antagonists, by several calcium antagonists and by some drugs acting on Ca^{2+} and Na^+ influx (Siesjo 1992b).

Acidosis arises as a result of sustained tissue ischaemia; it may contribute to tissue damage and prevent or retard recovery during reoxygenation by several mechanisms. When the ischaemia is sustained, acidosis may promote oedema formation by inducing Na^+ and Cl^- accumulation via coupled Na^+/H^+ and Cl^-/HCO^+ exchange; it may also prevent recovery of mitochondrial metabolism and resumption of H^+ extrusion (Siesjo 1992b). If the ischaemia is transient, pronounced intraischaemic acidosis triggers delayed damage characterised by gross oedema and seizures; possibly this is as a result of free radical formation. If the ischaemia is moderate, as in the penumbral zone of a focal ischaemic lesion, the effect of acidosis is controversial (Siesjo 1992b).

9.4 Free radicals and related molecules

Although free radicals have long been assumed to be mediators of ischaemic cell death, it is only recently that more convincing evidence of their role in ischaemia has been reported. A free radical is any atom, group of atoms, or molecules with an unpaired electron in its outermost orbital (Halliwell 1994). Since covalent chemical bonds usually consist of a pair of electrons sharing an orbital, free radicals can be thought of as molecules with an 'open' or 'half bond', and it is this which accounts for their extreme reactivity (Schmidley 1990). Free radicals are also produced in small amounts by several other mechanisms, including normal cellular processes, leaks in the mitochondrial transport system, reactions catalysed by prostaglandin hydroperoxidase, and by-products of the normal or pathological function of several other enzymes (Schmidley 1990; De Bono 1994).

Free radicals comprise aggressive oxygen species such as the superoxide anion radical, hydroxyl radical, hydrogen peroxide and singlet molecular oxygen. They damage DNA, proteins, carbohydrates and unsaturated lipids of all body compartments. Unfortunately, their direct investigation *in vivo* is difficult because most species have an extremely short half-life and cannot easily be studied under physiological conditions. Indirect evidence of increased free radical activity (oxidative damage) may be obtained by measurement of antioxidant concentrations in all tissue and body fluids. A state of increased oxidative damage by aggressive oxygen species implies insufficiency of the body's defence system (antioxidant concentration). Lines of defence against the damaging effects of free radicals consist of enzymes such as superoxide dismutase, catalase and glutathione peroxidase, non-essential endogenous radical scavengers (e.g. glutathione, albumin and other proteins, uric acid and ubiquinol-10) and essential radical scavengers such as the anti-oxidant vitamins including vitamin C (ascorbic acid), vitamin E (α-tocopherol) and the singlet oxygen-quenching carotenoids (e.g. β-carotene which is also a potential vitamin A precursor).

Several investigators have administered radical scavengers and extrapolated the presence of neurological protection afforded by these compounds as a measure of radical production. Other investigators have extrapolated changes that occur in endogenous radical scavengers as a measure of radical production. For example, α-tocopherol, ascorbic acid and reduced ubiquinones are endogenous substances which are thought to play important roles as chain breakers in radical reactions in the brain (Traystamn et al. 1991). During ischaemia there is a reduced concentration of ascorbic acid in brain parenchyma (Flamm et al. 1978); however, this may be attributable to a decrease in NADH-dependent recycling of ascorbic acid rather than increased utilisation by radical processes. During reperfusion, changes in lipid-soluble endogenous antioxidants (e.g. α-tocopherol and reduced ubiquinones), but not in water-soluble antioxidants such as ascorbic acid, are consistent with lipid peroxidation as an important mechanism of radical damage during reperfusion (Cooper et al. 1980; Yoshida et al. 1982).

Recently four different techniques for direct measurement of free radicals in brain have been described: nitroblue tetrazolium (NBT) reduction, chemiluminescence, electron spin resonance (ESR) spectroscopy and salicylate trapping (Imaizumi et al. 1984; Kontos at al. 1985; Armstead et al. 1988; Cao et al. 1988; Mirro et al. 1989).

9.5   Potential mechanisms for production of radicals during cerebral ischaemia

In normal mitochondrial respiration, cytochrome c is involved in four-electron transfer to reduce oxygen to water without production of oxygen radicals. During electron transport, the presence of oxygen at the terminal of the chain favours the maintenance of the members of the carrier system in an oxidised state.

When oxygen supply is limited during ischaemia, the electron transport chain of the inner mitochondrial membrane becomes highly reduced: in this reduced state, oxygen radicals may be produced. Studies in brain implicate the ubiquinone–cytochrome b region as the major site of oxygen radical production when mitochondria are in a maximally reduced state (Cino & Del Maestro 1989; Traystamn et al. 1991).

9.6 Potential mechanisms for production of radicals during reperfusion

When blood flow to the brain is disrupted, oxygen deprivation occurs, resulting in ischaemic conditions. With the resumption of blood flow, the subsequent reperfusion produces large quantities of superoxide radical and hydrogen peroxide. In addition, membrane lipids of the brain are very rich in polyunsaturated fatty acid chains, providing the perfect medium for lipid peroxidation (Halliwell 1989). The brain has very little catalase (the enzyme that converts hydrogen peroxide to H_2O and O_2), and diminished quantities of superoxide dismutase and glutathione peroxidase (another enzyme known to convert hydrogen peroxide and reduced glutathione to water and oxidised glutathione (Halliwell & Gutteridge 1985)).

Severe cerebral ischaemia is associated with failure of ATP-dependent ionic pumps; this results in the rapid loss of cellular potassium and influx of sodium, chloride and calcium (Siesjo 1984). Calcium influx during ischaemia may be involved in breakdown of lipid membrane through activation of phospholipase C and accumulation of free fatty acids (Wieloch & Siesjo 1982; Sun et al. 1984). Increase in arachidonic acid, in particular, may correlate with the duration of ischaemia (Shiu & Nemoto 1981), and levels are higher in brain regions that are more prone to damage after ischaemia and reperfusion (Westerberg et al. 1987). Accumulation of arachidonic acid may also produce cerebral oedema (Chan & Fishman 1980, 1987) and cause release of toxic neurotransmitters (Chan et al. 1983; Yu et al. 1986). Arachidonic acid accumulated during ischaemia is metabolised upon reperfusion via the lipoxygenase and cyclogenase pathways to produce prostaglandins, thromboxanes (Gaudet et al. 1980; Kempski et al. 1987) and superoxides (Armstead et al. 1988). Oxygen radicals may cause brain injury (Demopoulos et al. 1980) directly by lipid peroxidation (Yoshida et al 1980) and indirectly by vascular paralysis (Wei et al. 1985). Pre-treatment with cycloxygenase inhibitors can block the post-ischaemic accumulation of arachidonic acid metabolites (Gaudet et al. 1980), superoxide generation (Armstead et al. 1988), the delayed decrease in cerebral blood flow (Hallenbeck & Furlow 1979) and neurological deterioration (Chan & Fishman 1980). In addition to cycloxygenase-dependent superoxide production in brain tissues during reperfusion, oxygen radical production may also be related to the increase in pial arteriolar pressure which occurs with reperfusion (Armstead et al. 1988).

Toxic oxygen metabolites may also be produced during reperfusion through a mechanism that depends on the degradation of ATP. With the onset of ischaemia, brain adenine nucleotides are metabolised to nucleosides and purine bases with a rapid rise in the interstitial concentration of adenosine, which is further metabolised to inosine and hypoxanthine (Van Wylen et al.

1986). In the presence of oxygen, as occurs with reperfusion, metabolism of inosine and hypoxanthine via the xanthine oxidase pathway results in production of oxygen free radicals (Traystamn et al. 1991). Under normal circumstances, the brain has a low xanthine oxidase activity; however, during ischaemia and reperfusion, xanthine oxidase activity rises, and this may be important for superoxide production during reperfusion (Betz 1985).

Xanthine oxidase may be important in the formation of oxygen radicals during reperfusion in brain and some investigators have shown that blocking the enzyme activity may improve recovery from cerebral ischaemia and reperfusion (Patt et al. 1988). Allopurinol, which has the ability to cross the blood–brain barrier (Kim et al. 1987), has been found to inhibit xanthine oxidase when given in sufficient amounts and also to decrease infarct volume and improve neurological outcome after permanent focal ischaemia (Iansek et al. 1986; Martz et al 1989). However, allopurinol also has the ability to scavenge hydroxyl radicals; therefore its mechanism of protection may not be entirely due to its effect on xanthine oxidase (Moorhouse et al. 1987).

Another potential source of free radicals is the metabolism of arginine with the production of nitric oxide (Schmidt et al. 1988). In normal brain, nitric oxide appears to be non-toxic; however, during reperfusion and in the presence of superoxide, nitric oxide can potentially lead to the formation of hydroxyl radical-like reactive species (Beckman et al. 1990).

There is some evidence that leukocytes contribute to reperfusion injury in brain through release of chemotaxic factors and interaction with platelets to metabolise arachidonic acid and produce oxygen radicals (Hallenbeck et al. 1986; Kochanek et al. 1987).

9.7   Site and mediators of brain injury during radical production

Although both parenchyma and vascular endothelium have potential pathways for radical production, it is unclear which of these sites is the main source of radical production during reperfusion (Traystamn et al. 1991).

Free radical species of potential importance in cerebral ischaemia include the superoxide and hydroxyl group. The hydroxyl radical is the more reactive and more toxic of the two radicals. Hydrogen peroxide, while not a free radical *per se*, has the potential to generate hydroxyl radicals in reactions with superoxide, catalysed by iron. To function as a catalyst for this reaction, the iron must not be bound to proteins. Since the cerebrospinal fluid (CSF), unlike most extracellular fluids, has a low concentration of iron-binding proteins, iron released from damaged brain cells is more likely to be readily available to catalyse the generation of hydroxyl radicals.

Normally, the brain has efficient scavenging systems that maintain a low concentration of the factors necessary for these reactions to occur. However, in some models of ischaemia there is a decreased concentration of ascorbic acid and an increase in low molecular mass iron in the brain (Flamm et al. 1978; Traystamn et al. 1991).

Superoxide has been detected with the nitroblue tetrazolium (NBT) technique at the onset of reperfusion (Armstead et al. 1988). It is not as reactive as other radical species, but there is evidence that it is capable of causing primary injury in brain during ischaemia and reperfusion (Fridovich, 1986).

9.8   Mechanism of brain injury during radical production

Within the brain, oxygen radicals impair capillary endothelial cell mechanisms that help maintain homeostasis of electrolytes and water, and alter membrane fluidity characteristics (Lo & Betz 1986; Phelan & Lange 1990). Oxidative mechanisms also appear to contribute to synaptic damage within the brain (Pellmar & Neel 1989).

Most of the experimental work on free radicals in cerebral ischaemia has concentrated on damage to membrane lipids. Neuronal membranes are rich in polyunsaturated fatty acids which are particularly susceptible to free radical attack. There is consistent evidence that lipid peroxidation takes place when cerebral ischaemia is followed by reperfusion, and that lipid peroxidation depends on both adequate production of oxygen radicals and the presence of metal catalyst (iron) at the site where radicals are produced (Yoshida et al. 1980; Halliwell & Gutteridge 1984).

9.9   Therapeutic uses of radical scavengers

Several different radical scavengers and antioxidants have been tested for their efficacy in preventing biochemical, histological, physiological or neurological abnormalities after transient ischaemia. Kocaturk et al. (2001) examined copper/zinc superoxide dismutase (Cu/Zn-SOD) and catalase activities and copper and zinc concentrations, in both plasma and erythrocytes in cerebrovascular accident patients and a control group. The results showed that Cu/Zn-SOD activity was increased markedly in patients compared with the young controls, and reached a peak on day 5 of the disease, whereas the catalase activity of the patients on days 3 and 5 were in the normal range, but higher on day 10. The enzyme activities of the elderly group were generally increased compared with the young controls. Copper and zinc concentrations showed corresponding alterations. These findings suggest that the effects of oxidative stress in cerebrovascular accident might be reflected in erythrocyte and plasma parameters.

A research study which examined regional distribution and age-related change of SOD and nitric oxide synthase activities in the brain of stroke-prone spontaneously hypertensive rats, indicated that hypertensive vascular disease observed in these rats resulted from the decreased antioxidant capacity that is closely associated with the development of stroke and, in turn, shortened lifespan (Kimoto-Kinoshita et al. 1999).

The enzymes SOD and catalase are present naturally in brain; however, in the setting of ischaemia and reperfusion their capacity may be inadequate (White et al. 1985). The role of SOD is to scavenge superoxide and that of catalase is to scavenge hydrogen peroxide. In very high doses, intravenous administration of SOD has been shown to induce marked improvement in neurological recovery from acute hypertension and transient spinal cord ischaemia; however, in animals exposed to cerebral ischaemia and reperfusion, neurological recovery does not take place (Lim et al. 1986; Frosman et al. 1988; Zhang & Ellis 1990).

SOD has two drawbacks as a therapeutic agent. Firstly, it is readily cleared by the kidney and has a circulatory half-life of only 8 minutes in rats (Turrens et al. 1984). Secondly, Cu/Zn-SOD is a large water-soluble molecule and therefore cannot readily penetrate cell membranes or cross the blood–brain barrier in significant quantities after intravenous administration (Petkau et al. 1976). This is probably why it has only limited efficacy against reperfusion injury in the brain.

Conjugation of SOD to polyethylene glycol (PEG) monomers increases its circulatory half-life to almost 40 hours in rats (Wei et al. 1985). When the SOD–PEG combination was administered intravenously before transient ischaemia, infarct volume was decreased (Matsumiya et al. 1991). Liposomal entrapment has also been used successfully to decrease plasma clearance of SOD and increase its delivery to brain (Freeman et al. 1983).

Dimethyl sulphoxide is a hydroxyl radical scavenger which has been found to improve neurological outcome and reduce microscopic evidence of damage when given to animals just before reperfusion from spinal cord ischaemia (Coles et al. 1986).

The 21-aminosteroids are a group of compounds that lack classical steroid activities but are potent inhibitors of lipid perioxidation *in vivo*. The most extensively studied agent of this group in the setting of ischaemia and reperfusion is tirilazad. A 1996 report of a randomised double-blinded vehicle-controlled trial found that tirilazad mesylate (6 mg/kg per day for 3 days) administered beginning at a median of 4.3 hours after stroke did not improve outcome (RANTTAS Investigators 1996). Another study which used higher doses of tirilazad but was stopped prematurely by the sponsor for safety reasons reported a better outcome in the treated group at 3 months (Haley 1998).

9.10 Therapeutic potential of antioxidants and related substances

Until recently, little was known about the possible protective effect of anti-oxidants and their concentrations during and immediately following acute ischaemic stroke.

Although reactive oxygen species have long been assumed to be mediators of ischaemic cell death, it is only recently that convincing evidence of their role in ischaemia has been reported. Animal models of transient ischaemia and reperfusion in the brain suggest that brain lipids are vulnerable to oxidative attack during this period (Yoshida et al. 1980, 1984). There is some evidence that this effect is enhanced by poor α-tocopherol (vitamin E) status and can be mitigated by supplementation with this vitamin (Yamamoto et al. 1983; Yoshida et al. 1984). Similarly, experimental systems have provided evidence to suggest that oxidative mechanisms contribute to loss of membrane function and synaptic damage during ischaemia and reperfusion (Lo & Betz 1986; Pellmar & Neel 1989; Phelan & Lange 1990). A reduction in the tissue concentration of ascorbic acid (vitamin C) and α-tocopherol in cerebral ischaemia or during reperfusion is also suggestive of a role for these anti-oxidants *in vivo* (Flamm et al. 1978; Cooper et al. 1980; Yoshida et al. 1982). For example, the administration of α-tocopherol in membranes before the onset of ischaemia significantly reduced the levels of free radicals and lipid peroxides following reperfusion, and α-tocopherol may have had a protective role against the damage caused by cerebral ischaemia (Yamamoto et al. 1983). Likewise, if rats are raised on a diet deficient in α-tocopherol, exposure to ischaemia and reoxygenation results in enhanced lipid peroxidation (Yoshida et al. 1984).

De Keyser et al. (1992) studied serum concentrations of vitamins A and E in 80 patients with acute middle cerebral artery ischaemia within 24 hours of admission to hospital, and compared them with 80 controls matched for age and sex and who had various neurological disorders other than acute cerebral ischaemia. A high serum vitamin A concentration seemed to improve early outcome (within the first 21 days) of ischaemic stroke. A small uncontrolled study in humans found increased plasma levels of lipid hydroperoxides (markers of oxidative stress) in patients with ischaemic stroke (Polidori et al. 1998). An association between the plasma concentration of ascorbic acid and vitamin E and the degree of neurological impairment after ischaemic stroke was reported by Leinonen et al. (2000) who also demonstrated an association between plasma total antioxidant activity and the volume of ischaemic cerebral infarction and the degree of subsequent neurological impairment. Cherubini et al. (2000) also found evidence of reduced antioxidant concentrations in ischaemic stroke patients; higher vitamin A and uric acid concentrations but lower vitamin C levels and erythrocyte SOD activity were associated with poor early clinical outcome.

Ullegaddi et al. (2002) recently reported a pilot work in which 20 ischaemic stroke patients were randomly assigned to receive 800 IU (727 mg) of vitamin E and 500 mg of vitamin C orally, or no treatment, within 12 hours of stroke onset, and then once daily for 14 days. The results showed that supplementation of acute ischaemic stroke patients with vitamins E and C for 2 weeks significantly increased plasma concentrations of these vitamins and of total antioxidant capacity. Their study is still ongoing at the time of writing; however, further studies are needed to evaluate clinical benefits of such simple treatment in this group of patients.

9.11 Antioxidant capacity

An enhanced antioxidant capacity (individual and total) after acute stroke may protect against the adverse effects of free radicals produced during ischaemia and reperfusion. Total antioxidant capacity (TAC) of biological fluids is, however, regarded as more physiologically representative, in certain settings, than levels of individual antioxidants, and is believed to be a useful measure of the ability of antioxidant present in the fluids to protect against oxidative damage to membranes and other cellular components (Ryan et al. 1997).

An observational cohort study by Garibulla et al. (2002) of 31 acute ischaemic stroke patients, 26 hospitalised non-stroke patients and 23 community-based healthy controls recently examined changes in (individual and total) antioxidant capacity. Non-fasting venous blood was obtained within 24 hours, 48–72 hours and 7 days after stroke onset and hospitalisation for non-stroke patients, and at baseline for community controls; vitamins E and C, total plasma glutathione, TAC, uric acid, thiobarbituric acid reactive substances (TBARS), serum albumin, transferrin and C-reactive proteins (CRPs) were measured. Baseline glutathione concentrations were non-significantly lower and TBARS significantly higher in ischaemic stroke patients than in controls (Table 9.1); serum TAC strongly correlated with serum uric acid (Table 9.2, Figures 9.2 and 9.3)). In a multivariate analysis, serum uric acid explained most of the variance in total antioxidant capacity during the study period. Total antioxidant capacity was reduced in stroke patients, despite greater concentrations of uric acid than in controls (Table 9.3). Serum vitamin C concentrations deteriorated significantly in stroke patients, and differences between the cumulative changes between stroke patients and hospital controls were also statistically significant.

Indirect information on the impact of free radicals on the mechanism of brain injury may be obtained from comparison of antioxidant concentrations, because serious damage by free radicals implies insufficiency of the body's

Table 9.1 Baseline and follow-up markers of antioxidant capacity and oxidative stress in stroke patients and control groups [mean (SE)]. Reproduced from Gariballa et al. (2002) with permission from Oxford University Press.

Markers	Stroke patients (n = 31)			Hospital controls (n = 26)			Community controls (n = 23), baseline
	Baseline (24 h)	48–72 h	7 days	Baseline (24 h)	48–72 h	7 days	
Serum vitamin C[a] (μmmol/l)	39.0 (6)	33.3 (4)	32.1 (5)[b]	31.2 (4.9)	28.6 (5.8)	30.4 (6.3)[b]	66.6 (5.9)
Serum vitamin E (μmmol/l)	17.4 (1.7)	16.7 (1.5)	15.1 (1.0)	15.0 (0.9)	13.6 (1.3)	12.9 (0.8)	14.1 (1.1)
Plasma glutathione (μmmol/l)	0.18 (0.02)	0.17 (0.02)	0.19 (0.03)	0.22 (0.03)	0.23 (0.06)	0.21 (0.05)	0.35 (0.08)
TAC (μmmol/l)	540 (38)	516 (28)	487 (39)	550 (38)	545 (70)	603 (113)	568 (35)
TBARS[a] (μmmol/l)	5.64 (0.52)	5.08 (0.43)	5.90 (0.53)	5.27 (0.27)	5.57 (0.44)	4.52 (0.37)	4.26 (0.16)
Urate[a] (μmmol/l)	398 (20)	362 (21)	330 (22)	330 (25)	345 (47)	328 (50)	303 (35)
C-reactive proteins[a] (mg/l)	18.3 (5)	22.9 (7)	39.7 (10)[b]	63.4 (17)	70 (22)	33.1 (11)[b]	3.5 (0.7)

[a] One-way ANOVA for differences in baseline values between three groups and after adjusting for smoking, drug intake and CRPs (TBARS $P = 0.04$; urate $P = 0.05$; CRP $P = 0.001$).
[b] Mann–Whitney U-test for differences between the cumulative changes in stroke patients and hospital controls (vitamin C, $P = 0.01$, CRPs $P = 0.01$).

Table 9.2 Correlations between the total antioxidant capacity and uric acid concentration in serum of stroke patients and control groups [mean (SE)]. Reproduced from Gariballa et al. (2002) with permission from Oxford University Press.

	Stroke patients (n = 31)			Hospital controls (n = 26)			Community controls (n = 23), baseline
	Baseline (24 h)	48–72 h	7 days	Baseline (24 h)	48–72 h	7 days	
TAC (μmol/l)	540 (38)	516 (28)	487 (39)	550 (38)	545 (70)	603 (113)	568 (35)
Uric acid (160–400 μmol/l)	398 (20)	362 (21)	330 (22)	330 (25)	345 (47)	328 (50)	303 (35)
Correlation coefficient [r]	0.78[a]	0.79[a]	0.74[a]	0.87[a]	0.74[a]	0.86[a]	0.53[b]

[a] $P < 0.001$; [b] $P < 0.05$.
Results adjusted for CRPs

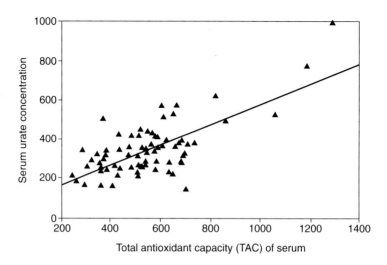

Figure 9.2 Correlation between baseline serum TAC and urate concentration for all patients and controls combined. Reproduced from Gariballa et al. (2002) with permission of Oxford University Press.

multilevel defence systems against radicals. A number of compounds present in serum have been shown to possess chain-breaking antioxidant capacity, in aqueous or organic solution *in vitro*, including vitamins C and E, albumin, urate, bilirubin and protein thiols (Gey et al. 1993a). This variety of components of serum with potential antioxidant capacity has led to the development

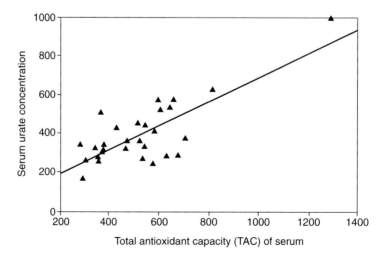

Figure 9.3 Correlation between baseline serum TAC and urate concentration for stroke patients. Reproduced from Gariballa et al. (2002) with permission of Oxford University Press.

Table 9.3 Multiple regression result for all subjects compared with stroke patients with baseline total antioxidant capacity as the dependent variable. Reproduced from Gariballa et al. (2002) with permission from Oxford University Press.

Variable/ independent predictor	R square		R square change		P value	
	All subjects	Strokes	All subjects	Strokes	All subjects	Strokes
Vitamin C	0.032	0.160	0.032	0.160	0.135	0.029*
Vitamin E	0.032	0.224	0.000	0.064	0.898	0.146
Glutathione	0.039	0.247	0.007	0.023	0.484	0.384
Uric acid	0.528	0.679	0.489	0.432	0.000*	0.000*
CRP	0.533	0.719	0.005	0.040	0.401	0.079
Albumin	0.533	0.725	0.000	0.007	0.824	0.453
Transferrin	0.533	0.730	0.000	0.005	0.962	0.548
Age	0.538	0.731	0.004	0.000	0.448	0.845

*$P < 0.05$.

and widespread use of assays which measure TAC, thereby providing clinically useful global measurements (Ryan et al. 1997). Ryan et al. (1997) also reported that in healthy subjects, TAC measured using enhanced chemiluminescence (ECL) is almost completely accounted for by uric acid, the end product of purine metabolism that has long been regarded as a potent endogenous water-soluble antioxidant and radical scavenger in humans (Becker 1993). However, its therapeutic benefit in diseases in which free radicals are thought to be involved is yet to be proven. There is some evidence that increased oxidative stress is associated with high circulating uric acid levels and that uric acid may protect against oxidative modification of endothelial enzymes and preserves the ability of endothelium to mediate vascular dilatation in the face of oxidative stress (Becker 1993). In contrast, there is some evidence that uric acid may have a direct role in the atherosclerotic process, because human atherosclerosis plaque contains more uric acid than do control arteries (Suarna et al. 1995). Following cerebral ischaemia and reperfusion, however, the metabolism of nucleosides and purine bases to inosine and hypoxanthine via the xanthine oxidase pathway results in production of oxygen free radicals (Traystamn et al. 1991; Patt et al. 1988) have shown that blocking the enzyme activity may improve recovery from cerebral ischaemia and reperfusion.

Waring (2002) reviewed the evidence on the role of uric acid as an antioxidant in acute ischaemic stroke. He reported that despite the widely held view that elevated serum uric acid concentrations confer increased risk of atherosclerotic disease, there is no compelling biological evidence of a causal link. Free radical activity is characteristically increased in patients with any one of several major cardiovascular risk factors, and is thought to play a key role in the early development of atherosclerosis. As an antioxidant, uric acid could be expected to confer protection against free radicals and, in the context of acute ischaemic stroke, there is growing evidence supporting its protective role. This underpins the importance of oxidative stress in the pathogenesis of acute stroke, and strengthens the rationale for further investigation of anti-oxidant treatments in this condition. The feasibility of uric acid administration to temporarily increase circulating concentrations has been established (Waring et al. 2001), and might allow its potential therapeutic impact to be examined in a clinical setting. Ongoing basic research is likely to shed new light on the cardiovascular effects of uric acid, and will hopefully allow the significance of serum concentrations to be interpreted more clearly.

Nevertheless, accepting the limitations of the present evidence, larger clin-ical studies in this area are needed to clarify the temporal relationships between antioxidant capacity and oxidative damage following ischaemia and reperfusion in man, and form the basis of appropriate antioxidant intervention strategies to minimise the long-term brain injury following cerebral ischaemia. Further work is also needed to explore the physiological roles of uric acid following acute ischaemic stroke.

9.12 Summary

There is strong indirect evidence that free radical production may be an important mechanism of brain injury after exposure to ischaemia and reperfusion, all of which may be associated with nutritional problems; if this is the case, the therapeutic rewards of obviating such problems may be great. The role of free radical formation in the pathogenesis of ischaemic brain damage and the neuroprotective effect of antioxidants are not defi-nitely established and need further study. There is also a need to develop and validate better techniques for direct measurement of antioxidant capacity and oxidative stress, and adjust for confounding variables. How-ever, the administration of antioxidants can give protective effects or worsen damage, depending on where in the sequence of events they are given.

10 Protein–Energy Undernutrition after Stroke

10.1 Introduction

Most studies report that food intake is less in hospital and institutionalised patients than in community-living elderly people (Department of Health and Social Security 1992). The reasons for this are likely to be a combination of poor food intake and extra demand due to the extra energy cost of metabolic disturbances associated with illness or disability. Ill health frequently has an adverse effect on nutritional status, especially in elderly people. For most people, these effects are limited to the time of acute illness, and the temporary nutritional disadvantage is overcome depending on the body reserves when the customary pattern of eating is resumed. However, if episodes of ill health occur repeatedly or become prolonged, nutritional status may decline step by step (Department of Health and Social Security 1992). For stroke patients, the fast phase of recovery takes several weeks, and slows down thereafter, but probably continues for at least 6 months in at least one-third of the survivors (Wade 1992). The overall metabolic requirements in the acute or long-term post-stroke period are not well described. It is possible, however, to extrapolate from data describing metabolic responses during injury and stress. For example, metabolic rates in patients with head injuries have been noted to increase to at least 140% of the predicted energy expenditure for a non-injured patient. In addition, protein degradation exceeds protein synthesis, with approximately 25% of available protein contributing to energy expenditure (Young et al. 1987; Buelow & Jamieson 1990).

10.2 Neurological deficit

Not all strokes produce the complete range of neurological deficit and there is an almost infinite range of possible combinations of loss of function; the more common ones include the following: disturbed level of consciousness (30–40%), difficulty in swallowing (30%), motor weakness (50–80%) or disturbance of sensory function (25%), slurred speech (30%), dysphasia/aphasia (30%) and visual field defects (7%) (Wade et al. 1985). These deficits will have a variable impact on a stroke patient's nutritional demands and actual intake.

For example, hemiplegia (paralysis of one half of the body) can affect nutritional intake in several ways. If a patient's dominant side is affected, they will have to use their non-dominant hand, which will make eating difficult and tedious. Motor movement and sensory input necessary for chewing and swallowing can also be affected in hemiplegia. During mastication, decreased sensation can cause pouching of food in the affected area without the patient being aware of it. Perceptual deficits, visual field defects and cognitive impairment together with motor apraxia can lead to decreased food intake and hence affect nutritional status. Dysphagia (difficulty in swallowing) has obvious implications for adequate nutritional intake. Gordon et al. (1987) demonstrated that dysphagia led to complications in 43% of first episode hemispheric stroke patients, 86% of whom were able to swallow normally 2 weeks later.

Immobility is another important factor that affects the nutritional status of stroke patients in several ways: (1) there are increased protein needs due to muscle wasting, (2) loss of calcium from bones, and (3) decubitus ulcers due to skin necrosis caused by excessive and prolonged pressure which lead to excess nitrogen losses from the patient. The negative nitrogen balance induced by immobility, in turn, increases the patient's susceptibility to further skin ulceration (Mahony 1973).

Equally or perhaps more important is the fact that assessment, recognition and treatment of malnutrition remain significant problems in hospital. This may be because nutritional assessment is not recognised as an integral part of a patient's clinical management; for stroke patients, one of the causes of their decreased nutritional intake is that the staff looking after them are not specifically trained to assess and meet their nutritional demands.

10.3   Eating problems following stroke

Although there are few who would argue against the importance of nutrition as part of stroke patients' short- and long-term management, the dietician is not often regarded as an integral member of the multidisciplinary team responsible for stroke management. Some studies have demonstrated that eating problems are common in stroke patients, and that the proportion of undernourished patients was higher on discharge than on admission (Axelsson et al. 1984, 1989).

Westergren et al. (2001) reported that of 162 stroke patients studied, 80% had eating difficulties and 52.5% were dependent on assisted eating.

10.4   Undernutrition following acute stroke

Patients suffering from acute stroke often face serious eating problems; this is likely to affect their nutritional status and possibly their short- and long-term outcome. Among patients with acute stroke, undernutrition was reported at a frequency of 16% on admission and 22% at discharge (Axelsson et al. 1988). Unosson et al. (1994) studied the nutritional status of 50 people consecutively admitted with stroke and aged 70 years or older; they found that low serum albumin and anergy were common and more so among those who were heavily dependent. A study by Davalos et al. (1996) of the nutritional status of 105 patients with acute stroke at admission and after 1 week reported that malnutrition was associated with increased stress reaction during the first week and was an important predictor of poor prognosis.

Recent new studies have been published which found that a high proportion of stroke patients had low anthropometric and biochemical values on admission. A study of 201 consecutive hospitalised stroke patients (Gariballa et al. 1998b) found that 99 (49%) had a triceps skin-fold thickness (TSF) below the 25th centile and 46 (23%) had a TSF below the 5th centile; 25 (12%) had a mid-arm circumference (MAC) below the 25th centile and four (2%) had a MAC below the 5th centile; 14% of the patients had arm muscle circumference (AMC) below the 25th centile and 3% below the 5th centile; 62 (31%) had a body mass index (BMI) of less than 20, and 38 (19%) had a serum albumin concentration below 35 g/1 (range 35–55 g/1). There were no significant differences in the nutritional status at admission between those who remained in hospital and the 'drop out' (early death or discharge) (Table 10.1). There were significant sex differences in some of the nutritional indices assessed on admission (Table 10.2). Undernutrition was evident in those who had lived in institutions or sheltered accommodation, but less so for those who lived in the

Table 10.1 Nutritional status at admission between stroke patients who remained in hospital for 4 weeks or more and the 'drop out' (early death or discharge). Reproduced from Gariballa et al. (1998b) with permission from *British Journal of Nutrition*.

Parameter[a]	Dropout (death and early discharge) (n = 150)		Stayed in hospital for 4 weeks or longer (n = 51)		95% CI	P value
	Mean	SD	Mean	SD		
BMI	22.5	4.6	22.4	4.3	−1.8 to 1.5	0.869
Body weight (kg)	64	13.5	62	13.9	−7.5 to 2.0	0.257
TSF (mm)	7.4	1.8	7.6	1.9	−1.3 to 2.4	0.381
BSF (mm)	5.0	1.5	5.0	1.7	−0.7 to 1.2	0.456
MAC (cm)	25.5	3.0	25.8	3.9	0.8 to 1.4	0.589
AMC (cm)	22.7	2.7	22.6	3.2	−1.0 to 0.9	0.465
Albumin (range 35–55 g/l)	38.2	3.6	38.1	3.7	−1.2 to 1.0	0.561
Transferrin (range 2–4 g/l)	2.8	0.6	2.8	0.8	−0.2 to 0.2	0.104
Iron (range 14–28 μmol/l)	9.4	0.8	8.8	0.7	−2.3 to 1.0	0.421

[a] AMC, arm muscle circumference; BMI, body mass index; BSF, biceps skin-fold thickness; MAC, mid-arm circumference; TSF, triceps skin-fold thickness.

Table 10.2 Nutritional status of men and women on admission. Reproduced from Gariballa et al. (1998b) with permission from *British Journal of Nutrition*.

Parameter[a]	Men (n = 87)		Women (n = 114)		Mean difference between men and women	95% CI	P value
	Mean	SD	Mean	SD			
BMI	22.2	3.9	22.9	5	−0.7	−2.2 to 0.8	0.335
Body weight (kg)	68	12.5	59.9	13.4	8.2	3.9 to 12.5	0.0001
TSF (mm)	5.7	1.6	9	1.9	−4.6	−6.1 to −3.1	0.0001
BSF (mm)	5.0	1.5	4.9	1.7	−0.3	−1.2 to 0.6	0.505
MAC (cm)	26.2	2.6	25.2	3.8	1.1	0.1 to 2.0	0.019
AMC (cm)	24.3	2.2	21.5	2.7	2.7	2.0 to 3.5	0.0001
Albumin (range 35–55 g/l)	38.8	3.5	37.9	3.8	1.0	−0.1 to 2.0	0.056
Transferrin (range 2–4 g/l)	2.66	0.45	2.83	0.77	−0.2	−0.4 to 0.02	0.084
Iron (range 14–28 μmol/l)	10.6	0.6	8.4	0.7	2.2	0.6 to 3.8	0.016
Haemoglobin (g/dl)	14.4	1.7	13.3	1.7	1.1	0.6 to 1.6	0.0001
Vitamin B12 (range 200–950 ng/l)	516	1.56	573	1.7	−56	−2.46 to 588	0.395
Serum folate (range 2.5–13 μg/l)	6.12	1.4	6.11	1.5	−0.2	−1.4 to 0.9	0.561

[a] For abbreviations, see Table 10.1.

community alone or with a spouse before admission; however, after adjusting for age the differences were not statistically significant (Table 10.3).

During the hospital stay, all measures of nutritional status except serum iron showed significant and marked deterioration over the study period (Table 10.4), with the most dramatic deterioration in nutritional status being seen in the first 2 weeks. Thus, within the first 2 weeks of hospitalisation 61 (64%) of those patients who survived lost weight, 29 (30%) gained weight and in 6 (6%) body weight remained unchanged to within 0.4 kg compared with 23 (45%), 24 (47%) and 5 (8%), respectively, during the second 2 weeks of the hospital stay. Nutritional status deteriorated significantly during the hospital stay for those who had lived in institutions or sheltered accommodation, but less so for those who had lived in the community alone or with a spouse (Table 10.5). Men lost more body weight than women during the course of hospitalisation, and their serum albumin showed significant deterioration compared with that of women at 4 weeks (Table 10.6). All measures of nutritional status with the exception of body weight showed a non-significant deterioration in those with a swallowing difficulty compared with those without (Table 10.7). Drug intake did not influence the nutritional status either on admission or during the hospital stay (Gariballa et al. 1998b).

During the study (Gariballa et al. 1998b), the dietician and nursing staff

Table 10.3 Nutritional status of stroke patients according to their residence in the community before admission. Reproduced from Gariballa et al. (1998b) with permission from *British Journal of Nutrition*.

Parameter[a]	Living with a spouse (n = 80)		Living alone (n = 67)		Living in insitution or sheltered accommodation (n = 51)		P value[b]
	Mean	SD	Mean	SD	Mean	SD	
Age	74	9	80	8	81	10	0.0001
Gender male (no., %)	56 (70)		24 (46)		25 (49)		0.0001
BMI	22.6	4.6	22.4	5.5	21.3	5.7	0.692
Body weight (kg)	66	14.8	62.8	12.4	60.4	11.9	0.486
MAC (cm)	26.4	3.4	25.5	3.4	24.6	3.1	0.399
AMC (cm)	23.6	3.0	22.1	2.6	21.8	2.7	0.051
TSF (mm)	7.1	1.8	8.1	1.9	7.2	1.9	0.189
BSF (mm)	5.1	1.5	4.8	1.6	4.9	1.7	0.448
Albumin (g/l)	38.6	3.8	38.1	3.7	37.8	3.6	0.831
Transferrin (g/l)	2.7	0.5	2.9	0.8	2.6	0.6	0.035
Iron (μmol/l)	9.8	0.95	9.5	0.64	8.3	0.55	0.667
Haemoglobin (g/dl)	13.9	1.9	13.8	1.9	13.4	1.6	0.523

[a] For abbreviations, see Table 10.1.
[b] P value for the main effects of residence on nutritional status indices after adjusting for age.

Table 10.4 Stroke patients (n = 51) who remained in hospital during the study period for whom complete nutritional measurements were obtained. Reproduced from Gariballa et al. (1998b) with permission from *British Journal of Nutrition*.

Parameter[a]	Week 0		Week 2		Week 4		P value
	Mean	SD	Mean	SD	Mean	SD	
BMI	22.51	4.5	21.4	4.4	21.65	4.1	0.006
Body weight (kg)	62.7	13.6	61.4	13.2	61.6	12.5	0.026
TSF (mm)	9.3	1.7	8.1	1.8	6.7	1.7	0.0001
BSF (mm)	5.7	1.6	4.9	1.5	4.2	1.5	0.0001
MAC (cm)	25.8	3.4	25.2	3.7	25.2	3.4	0.001
Albumin (range 35–55 gl)	38.0	3.8	35.5	4.2	34.8	4.0	0.0001
Transferrin (range 2–4 g/l)	2.76	0.65	2.61	0.58	2.6	0.47	0.023
Iron (range 14–28 μmol/l)	9.6	0.74	8.9	0.72	8.7	0.53	0.893

[a] For abbreviations, see Table 10.1.

Table 10.5 Serum albumin profile during the hospital stay of stroke patients according to their residence in the community before admission. Reproduced from Gariballa et al. (1998) with permission from *British Journal of Nutrition*.

Residence in community before admission	Serum albumin (g/l)					
	Week 0		Week 4		Mean change	95% CI
	Mean	SD	Mean	SD		
Living with a spouse (n = 32)	38.6	3.7	35.3	3.8	2.9	1.2–4.6
Living alone (n = 22)	38.1	3.7	34.9	4.5	2.6	1.3–3.9
Living in institution or sheltered accommodation (n = 18)	37.8	3.6	33.8	5.2	4.1	2.2–6.0

observed that many stroke patients made unsuitable food choices from the menus due to lack of supervision and assistance, which might have led to their nutritional intake being compromised. Because of their physical disability, stroke patients required assistance and a much longer time to finish their meals, something which is often cut short to fit in with the busy schedules of nursing staff.

In another study (Gariballa et al. 1998c), it was found that stroke patients with hypoalbuminaemia ($< 35 \, g/l$) had an increased risk of infective complications and poor functional outcome during hospitalisation compared with those with normal or higher serum concentrations. Serum albumin concentrations were good predictors of the degree of disability and handicap during the hospital stay (Table 10.8); after adjusting for poor prognostic indicators, the serum albumin concentration in hospital was a strong and independent predictor of mortality at 3 months following acute stroke (Gariballa et al. 1998c) {Tables 10.9, 10.10; Figures 10.1–10.3).

Choi-Kwon et al. (1998) studied the nutritional status of 88 female patients with first-ever strokes and 120 age-matched controls using three biochemical and five anthropometric measures. Strokes were divided into cerebral infarction ($n = 67$) and intracerebral haemorrhage ($n = 21$). The results suggested that undernutrition is prevalent in acute stroke patients, significantly more so in patients with intracerebral haemorrhage than in those with cerebral infarction, but the authors acknowledged that this study has a number of limitations and its results should be interpreted with caution.

Very recently, the results of an observational multicentre study of the relationship between baseline nutritional status and clinical outcome at 6 months in 2955 hospitalised stroke patients were published (FOOD Trial Collaboration 2003). Baseline nutritional status was independently associated with clinical

Table 10.6 Cumulative changes in nutritional variables of men and women measured fortnightly after hospital admission. Reproduced from Gariballa et al. (1998b) with permission from *British Journal of Nutrition*.

Parameter[a]	Week 2		Week 4			Week 2		Week 4		
	Mean	SD	Mean	SD	Net change	Mean	SD	Mean	SD	Net change
Number of patients	44		23			52		28		
BMI	−0.5	0.7	0.0	3.9	−0.5	−1.1	0.7	−0.2	3.2	−1.3
Body weight (kg)	−1.4	2.4	−0.2	1.7	−1.6	−2.0	2	0.9	1.8	−1.1
TSF (mm)	−0.5	1.1	−0.4	1.3	−0.9	−0.4	1.2	−1.03	1.4	−1.43
MAC (cm)	−0.7	1.7	0.8	1.1	0.1	−0.2	1.5	−0.2	1.2	−0.4
Albumin (g/l)[b]	−2.1	3.3	−2.2	2.8	−4.3	−2.6	3.6	−0.1	3.1	−2.7
Transferrin (g/l)	−0.06	0.6	0.01	0.4	−0.05	−0.1	0.6	−0.13	0.4	−0.23
Iron (μmol/l)	0.0	0.5	−1.3	0.6	−1.3	−0.5	0.6	0.6	0.7	0.1

[a] For abbreviations, see Table 10.1
[b] $P = 0.03$ for the difference between the cumulative changes in serum albumin levels in men and women.

Table 10.7 Nutritional status in stroke patients according to their ability to swallow on admission. Reproduced from Gariballa et al. (1998b) with permission from *British Journal of Nutrition*.

Parameter[a]	Able to swallow				Unable to swallow			
	Week 0		Week 2		Week 0		Week 2	
	Mean	SD	Mean	SD	Mean	SD	Mean	SD
Number of patients	178		83		23		13	
Body weight (kg)	64.1	13.3	62.8	13.3	60.7	15.5	60.5	16.6
MAC (cm)	25.7	3.2	25.4	3.3	24.4	3.4	23.5	3.9
TSF (mm)	7.6	1.9	7.1	1.9	6.6	1.7	5.7	1.4
Albumin (g/l)[b]	38.1	3.7	36.3	4.0	37.8	4.1	33.4	4.1
Transferrin (g/l)	2.8	0.7	2.7	0.6	2.5	0.5	2.4	0.6

[a] For abbreviations, see Table 10.1.
[b] $P = 0.0001$ for the difference in serum albumin levels in each group separately during the hospital stay, but $P > 0.05$ for the difference between the changes in the two groups.

Table 10.8 Spearman's rank correlation coefficients of serum albumin levels and functional outcome scores of stroke patients during hospitalisation. Reproduced from Gariballa et al. (1998c) with permission of the *American Journal of Clinical Nutrition*. © American Society for Clinical Nutrition.

Parameter[a]	Week 0	Week 2	Week 4
No. of patients	192	97	46
Serum albumin (g/l)	Median (Q1–39 (36–41) Q3)[b]	37 (34–39)	35 (33–38)
Barthel score	Median (Q1–37 (10–60) Q3)[b]	45 (15–70)	45 (26–70)
	R[c] 0.31[d]	0.49[d]	0.48[e]
Rankin score	Median (Q1–5 (4–6) Q3)[b]	4 (3–6)	4 (3–5)
	R[c] −0.28[d]	−0.46[d]	−0.47[e]
Orpington score	Median (Q1–4 (2.8–5.2) Q3)[b]	3.6 (2.4–4.8)	3.6 (2.8–4)
	R[c] −0.29[d]	−0.52[d]	−0.41[f]

[a] The Barthel scores ten functions on a scale 0 (fully dependent) to 20 or 100 (independent); for assessing disability it is more reliable and less subjective than other scores, so is less likely to be operator dependent. The original Rankin score was a five-point rating score that graded patients on their overall level of independence with reference to previous activities; its reliability in terms of inter-observer agreement and reproducibility has been evaluated with satisfactory results. The Orpington score was derived from a multivariate analysis of determinants of functional outcome in 96 stroke patients over 75 years of age. The score ranges from 1.6 (best prognosis) to 6.8 (worst prognosis).
[b] Q1–Q3, inter-quartile range.
[c] R, correlation coefficient.
[d] $P < 0.0001$.
[e] $P < 0.001$.
[f] $P < .0.01$.

outcome. The authors were able to study and follow up a large sample of stroke patients recruited from a wide range of hospitals from around the world, which does increase the external validity of the results. They used a simple bedside method, performed by the randomising clinician, to categorise patients as 'undernourished, normal or overweight' (60% of patients) or, where practical, a fuller assessment of nutritional status. Nine per cent of those enrolled were judged undernourished and 16% as overweight; undernutrition was associated with poor outcome.

Table 10.11 lists trials studying the prevalence of undernutrition in stroke patients in acute care settings and its influence on outcome.

Table 10.9 The Cox's proportional hazard analysis of the relationship between serum albumin and other independent variables on admission, and stroke patients' mortality. Reproduced from Gariballa et al. (1998c) with permission of the *American Journal of Clinical Nutrition*. © American Society for Clinical Nutrition.

Variable	P value	Hazard ratio for unit change	95% CI
Modified Rankin score (0–5)	0.002	1.63	1.20–2.22
Age (years)	0.003	1.06	1.02–1.10
Serum albumin (g/l)	0.030	0.91	0.84–0.99
Previous illnesses[a]	0.942	1.01	0.76–1.35
Drugs[a]	0.921	1.01	0.83–1.22
Smoking[b]	0.311	1.27	0.80–2.02
Gender	0.238	1.44	0.79–2.63

[a] Drug intake (2.7 drugs/person) and history of any previous illness (1.7 disease/person) on admission.
[b] Current = 1, Ex = 2.

Table 10.10 Survival analysis of stroke patients at 3 months according to serum albumin levels on admission, and after 2 and 4 weeks in hospital. Reproduced from Gariballa et al. (1998b) with permission of the *American Journal of Clinical Nutrition*. © American Society for Clinical Nutrition.

	Albumin (g/l)	Total number of patients	Number of deaths	Number alive	Proportion surviving (%)
Week 0[a]	≥ 35	160	34	126	78.75
	< 34	38	21	17	44.74
Week 2[b]	≥ 35	98	15	83	84.69
	< 34	47	27	20	42.55
Week 4[c]	≥ 35	42	4	38	90.48
	< 34	30	17	17	56.67

[a] $P < 0.0001$.
[b] $P < 0.0001$.
[c] $P = 0.0012$.

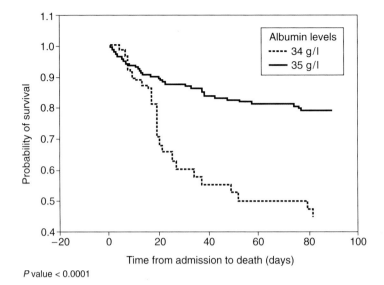

P value < 0.0001

Figure 10.1 Survival probability of stroke patients according to admission serum albumin. Reproduced from Gariballa et al. (1998c) with permission from *American Journal of Clinical Nutrition*. © American Society for Clinical Nutrition.

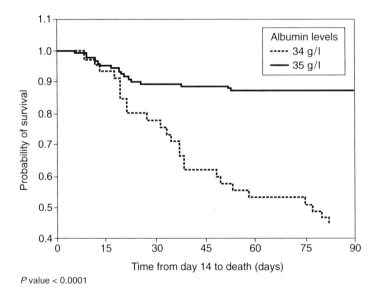

P value < 0.0001

Figure 10.2 Survival probability of stroke patients according to serum albumin at week 2. Reproduced from Gariballa et al. (1998c) with permission from *American Journal of Clinical Nutrition*. © American Society for Clinical Nutrition.

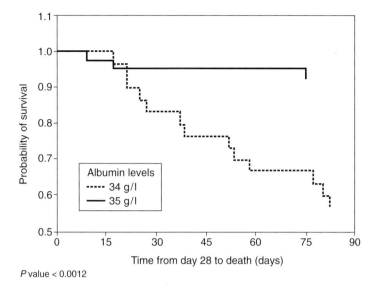

P value < 0.0012

Figure 10.3 Survival probability of stroke patients according to serum albumin at week 4. Reproduced from Gariballa et al. (1998c) with permission from *American Journal of Clinical Nutrition*. © American Society for Clinical Nutrition.

10.5   Nutrition status and demands during stroke rehabilitation

Nutritional depletion during rehabilitation may be more serious than during acute illness, since rehabilitation periods may extend over weeks and months, and loss of body weight, although less marked than in the early catabolic phase, may be greater overall. As long ago as 1971, Evans and Stock drew attention to the relative neglect of the nutritional problems of rehabilitation patients. When they compared nutrient intakes of long-stay, acutely ill and rehabilitation patients, they showed energy and protein intakes to be the lowest in the last group. Subsequent studies of the nutritional status and energy intake of 350 randomly selected admissions, including stroke patients, to a geriatric rehabilitation unit (Sullivan & Walls 1994; Sullivan et al. 1995) showed that protein–energy undernutrition (PEU) was a strong predictor of in-hospital mortality and was also a strong independent risk factor for one-year post discharge mortality. Furthermore, serum albumin as a clinical marker of PEU has been found to predict outcome in acute and non-acute stroke care settings (Aptaker et al. 1994; Sullivan et al. 1995).

Table 10.11 Prevalence of protein–energy undernutrition after acute stroke. From Gariballa (2000). Reproduced with permission from *British Journal of Nutrition*.

Authors & country	Participants	Sample size	Age mean (SD) (years)	Mean LOS[b] (SD) (days)	Time of assessments	Measures of nutritional status[a]	Definition of undernutrition	End-points	Comments
Axelsson et al. 1988 Sweden	Consecutive acute stroke patients admitted to a stroke unit	100 (64 males)	71 (8)	13.6	Within 4 days of admission and weekly thereafter	TSF, MAC, body weight, serum albumin, transferrin, and prealbumin	Two or more nutritional measures below normal values obtained from healthy population in Sweden	Nutritional status and related variables	16 (16%) patients undernourished on admission compared with 18 (22%) on discharge. Undernutrition appeared to be related to infections, male sex, intake of cardiovascular drugs and high age
Unosson et al. 1994 Sweden	Acute stroke patients admitted to a neurological unit	50 (23 males)	79 (4)	13.8 (6.5)	Within 48 hours of admission and after 2 and 9 weeks	Weight index, TSF, MAC, serum proteins (albumin, transthyretin and antitrypsin), delayed hypersensitivity, body composition (bioelectric impedance) and functional status	If at least three were lower than the following values (including one anthropometric, serum protein and skin test) Cut-off values for men and women, respectively, were as follows: weight index < 80% & < 80%; TSF, ≤ 6 mm & ≤12 mm; MAC, ≤23 cm & ≤19 cm in those aged ≤79 years and ≤21 cm & ≤18 cm in those aged > 79 years; transthyretin, <0.20 g/l & < 0.18 g/l; albumin, 36 g/l & 36 g/l; skin test, < 10 mm & < 10 mm.	Nutritional status and dependency	On admission four patients were undernourished. Low serum albumin and anergy were common among stroke patients with a severely impaired functional condition. Immobility leads to loss of body mass
Davlos et al. 1996 Spain	Consecutive stroke patients of less than 24 hour duration after the stroke	105 (67 males)	66 (10)	21 (16)	Within 24 hours of admission and weekly during the hospital stay	TSF, MAC, serum albumin and calorimetry	Values for each variable were expressed as a percentage of the 50th centile, adjusted for age and sex of a large sample of a healthy population living in the area	Nutritional status, morbidity and death	16.3% of patients were undernourished at inclusion and 26.4% after the first week. Undernourished patients showed higher stress reaction and increased frequency of infections. Undernutrition after 1 week was independently associated with increased risk of disability or death within 30 days of follow-up

Reference	Patients	N	Age	Timing	Measurements	Comparison	Outcome	Results
Gariballa et al. 1998b UK	Consecutive acute stroke patients	201 (81 males)	77.9 (9)	Within 48 hours of admission and after 2 and 4 weeks	Median (interquartile range) 23 (12–49)	Body weight, TSF, BSF, MAC, AMC, albumin, transferrin, iron, vitamin B12 and folate	Results compared with normal values standardised for age & sex from South Wales (Burr & Philips 1984)	Nutritional status and mortality	On admission 31% had BMI < 20; 49% had TSF < 25th centile; 12% had MAC < 25th centile and 19% had albumin <35 g/l. Baseline and in-hospital poor nutritional status were associated with poor clinical outcome
Gariballa et al. 1998c UK	Consecutive acute stroke patients	225 (96 males)	77.6 (9)	Within 48 hours of admission and after 2 and 4 weeks	Median (interquartile range) 23 (12–49)	Body weight, TSF, BSF, MAC, AMC, albumin, transferrin and iron	Results compared with normal values standardised for age and sex from South Wales (Burr & Philips 1984)	Morbidity and mortality	After adjusting for poor prognostic indicators (age, stroke severity and co-morbidity) low serum albumin at admission and during the hospital stay was a strong and independent predictor of death at 3 months after acute stroke. It also predicted poor functional status and increased morbidity
FOOD Trial Collaboration 2003 UK	Any stroke patient admitted to a participating hospital if the responsible clinician is uncertain of the best feeding policy	2955 (50% males)	73.3 (12)	At admission (within 7 days of the stroke)	Simple bedside method performed by randomising clinician (60% of patients) or, where practical, a fuller assessment of nutritional status	Patients were categorised as 'under-nourished, normal or overweight'	Morbidity and mortality at 6 months following the stroke	Undernutrition immediately after stroke was associated with reduced survival, functional ability and living circumstances at 6 months following the stroke; the relationship, although weakened when adjusted for other prognostic factors, remained statistically significant

[a] For abbreviations, see Table 10.1

[b] LOS, length of stay.

10.6 Summary

Stroke patients are probably the most vulnerable and are more likely than others to suffer from undernutrition during their hospital stay. A significant number are undernourished on admission and their nutritional status deteriorates further whilst in hospital. Undernutrition is associated with increasing morbidity and mortality during the hospital stay and subsequent discharge into the community.

11 Nutritional Status of Special Stroke Groups: Patients with Urinary Incontinence and Swallowing Difficulties

Despite urinary incontinence being such an important prognostic factor in the acute stage of stroke, there are many gaps in our knowledge of causes of poor outcome in incontinent stroke patients (Nakayama et al. 1997; Brittain et al. 1998). There are, however, well established predictors of poor outcome in hospitalised acute stroke patients, such as undernutrition, dehydration and infections, which are potentially treatable (Davalos et al. 1996; Gariballa et al. 1998b, c). A recent study of 215 consecutive stroke patients with complete records attempted to measure the influence of urinary incontinence on clinical outcome and to identify the contribution of potentially treatable factors such as undernutrition to stroke outcome (Gariballa 2002). After adjusting for the stroke severity, age and co-morbidity (chronic illness, drugs and smoking), urinary incontinence at admission was a significant predictor of stroke death at 3 months (Table 11.1).

The association between urinary incontinence and stroke mortality was still statistically significant, even after adjusting for a different set of variables including age, level of consciousness, sitting balance and motor power. Survival analysis of stroke patients for time of death according to continence status on admission demonstrated a significant relationship (Table 11.2). Figure 11.1 shows Kaplan–Meier survival curves for stroke patients within the first 3 months; those incontinent of urine had an increased risk of dying within the first 3 months following the stroke compared with those who were continent. Stroke patients incontinent of urine at admission were older, more disabled, undernourished and dehydrated compared with those who were continent (Table 11.3). During the hospital stay the nutritional status of incontinent stroke patients deteriorated significantly compared with continent patients (Table 11.3). During the hospital stay, 34 stroke patients incontinent of urine had 82 documented infective complications (2.4 infective episodes per patient) compared with 94 patients without incontinence who had 36 infective complications (0.4 infective episode per patient), $P < 0.001$.

Table 11.1 Cox's proportional hazard analysis of the relationship between urinary incontinence and other prognostic variables on admission and stroke patients' mortality. From Gariballa (2002).

Variable	Regression coefficient	Standard error	P value	Hazard ratio for unit change	95% CI
Age (years)	0.0724	0.0187	0.001	1.08	1.04–1.12
Modified Rankin score (0–5)	0.3817	0.1734	0.028	1.5	1.04–2.06
Urinary incontinence	1.0266	0.3732	0.006	2.8	1.30–5.80
Previous illnesses[a]	0.0507	0.1383	0.714	1.05	0.80–1.38
Drugs[a]	0.0231	0.0947	0.807	1.02	0.85–1.23
Smoking[b]	−0.1778	0.2306	0.441	1.19	0.76–1.90

[a] Drug intake (drugs/person) and history of previous illness (cerebrovascular accident, hypertension, ischaemic heart disease, heart failure, peripheral vascular disease, diabetes and atrial fibrillation), (disease/person) on admission.
[b] Never = 0, Ex = 1, Current = 2.

Table 11.2 Survival analysis[a] of stroke patients at 3 months according to continence status within 72 hours of admission to hospital. From Gariballa (2002).

	Total number of patients	Number of deaths	Number alive	Proportion surviving (%)
Continent	123	13	110	89
Incontinent	92	45	47	51.1

[a] Test statistics: log rank 42.19; $P < 0.001$.

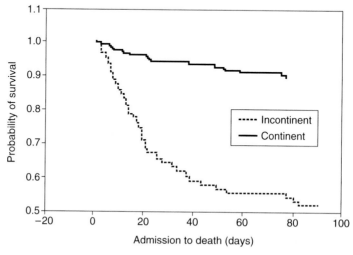

Significant difference in survival between continent and incontinent patients, $P < 0.001$

Figure 11.1 Survival curve for stroke patients (Kaplan–Meier) according to continence status at admission. Reproduced from Gariballa (2002).

Table 11.3 Nutritional status of stroke patients during hospital stay according to continence status. From Gariballa (2002).

	Continent of urine						Incontinent of urine					
	Week 0 (n = 123)		Week 2 (n = 58)		Week 4 (n = 30)		Week 0 (n = 92)		Week 2 (n = 45)		Week 4 (n = 19)	
	Mean	SD	Mean	SD	Mean	SD	Mean	SD	Mean	SD	Mean	SD
Age (years)	75.8	9.6					80.3	8.7				
Female gender (no., %)	69	55					59	64				
Body weight[a,b] (kg)	65.1	13	64.6	13	66.1	12	60.2	14	58.5	15	57	15
TSF[c] (mm)	9.0	5.7	8.1	5	7.3	4	9.0	6	8.4	5.7	8.5	5
MAC[d] (cm)	26.1	3	25.8	3.5	25.8	3.1	25	3.9	24.5	4	24.2	3.8
Albumin[a,b] (range 35–55 g/l)	39.3	3.2	37.3	3.6	35.8	3.3	36.7	3.7	34.5	4.3	34	4.6
Transferrin[a] (range 2–4 g/l)	2.90	0.7	2.83	0.6	2.70	0.5	2.60	0.6	2.42	0.5	2.46	0.5
Iron (range 14–28 mmol/l)	11.8	5.3	11.2	5	9.8	4.7	7.5	4.4	7.7	4.8	8.7	3.8

[a] $P \leq 0.05$ for within-subjects difference.
[b] $P \leq 0.05$ for between-subjects difference.

This study indicates that the poor outcome associated with urinary incontinence after acute stroke may partly be due to potentially modifiable risk factors such as undernutrition, dehydration and infections. Whether adequate hydration, nutritional supplementation and control of infections remove or mitigate the hazard of poor outcome associated with urinary incontinence following acute stroke needs to be determined. In the meantime, urinary incontinence in acute stroke patients may be used as one of the criteria for selecting patients for intensive treatment.

11.2   Nutritional status of dysphagic stroke patients

Dysphagia (difficulty in swallowing) has obvious implications for adequate nutritional intake; it was shown to complicate 43% of first episode hemispheric stroke cases, 86% of whom were able to swallow normally 2 weeks later (Gordon et al. 1987).

At present, it is not known how much poor intake of food contributes to the poor outcome which often follows insertion of a percutaneous endoscopic gastrostomy tube (PEG-tube), and whether improving the nutritional status before PEG-tube insertion would influence the outcome. However, it could also be argued that the association of increased complications and PEG-tube insertion in stroke patients results from patient selection, where those who need a PEG-tube are those with the poorest prognosis. This important area is in need of urgent research. The FOOD Trial Collaboration (2003), a large multi-centre study set up to evaluate various feeding policies in patients admitted to hospital with a recent stroke, reported that poor nutritional status on admission was associated with poor outcome. The recent Cochrane Database Systematic Review (Bath et al. 2002) of the effect of different management strategies for dysphagic stroke patients, in particular how and when to feed, whether to supplement nutritional intake, and how and whether to treat dysphagia reported that few studies have been performed, and these have involved too few patients. PEG-tube feeding may improve outcome and nutrition compared with nasogastric tube feeding. However, further research is required to assess how and when patients are fed, and the effect of stimulating swallowing by any means on dysphagia.

11.3   Ethical aspects of PEG-tube insertion in dysphagic stroke patients

The decision to place a PEG-tube in a dysphagic stroke patient focuses mainly on the patient's inability to take food by mouth. Clearly, many stroke patients who receive PEG-tubes are severely disabled and some may be in the terminal phase of their illness, raising the question of the appropriateness of the intervention. Recent guidelines for PEG-tube insertion suggest that for patients who have dysphagia without other deficits in quality of life, physicians should offer and recommend the procedure. For the remaining patients who have dysphagia with other deficits in quality of life, the physician's role is to provide non-directive counselling regarding the short- and long-term consequences of a trial of PEG-tube feeding (Rabeneck et al. 1997). As the majority of dysphagic stroke patients will have other deficits, it is therefore the treating doctor's duty to undertake adequate consultation with competent patients, closest relatives and all members of the multidisciplinary team involved with the patient before recommending the procedure. Considering the long-term implications of the PEG-tube after hospital discharge, the patient's social circumstances, quality of life and prognosis also have to be taken into account (Lennard-Jones 1999).

11.4 Summary

The poor outcome associated with swallowing difficulties and incontinence of urine after acute stroke may partly be due to potentially modifiable risk factors such as undernutrition, dehydration and infections. Whether adequate hydration, nutritional supplementation and control of infections remove or mitigate the hazard of poor outcome associated with swallowing difficulties and urinary incontinence following acute stroke needs to be determined. In the meantime, urinary incontinence and swallowing difficulties in acute stroke patients may be used as some of the criteria for selecting patients for intensive treatment.

12 Undernutrition after Acute Stroke: When Does it Matter?

12.1 Introduction

Distinguishing underlying disease from undernutrition, and to separate their effects on the ageing patient's outcome, is still a challenge for clinicians. This is because, (a) there is no universally accepted definition of undernutrition, (b) all current assessment parameters are affected by age-related changes, disability, illness and injury, (c) it is widely appreciated that the findings associated with underlying disease can confound detection of undernutrition and vice versa, and that either improvement or deterioration in one influences the other (Klein et al. 1997; Weinsier & Heimberger 1997).

During infection and injury a series of metabolic events are activated that lead to a state of negative nitrogen balance and significant loss of lean body mass (LBM). This process is mediated by inflammatory cytokines and is characterised by marked anorexia and net whole body protein breakdown (Chang & Bistrian 1997). The loss of lean body mass, if significant, may lead to adverse clinical outcome. Attempts to block the action of known cytokines did not normalise protein breakdown (Chang & Bistrian 1997). Two studies have demonstrated that the ability to replenish LBM with nutritional therapy may depend on the cause of LBM loss (Shike et al. 1984; Kotler et al. 1985). For example, when the loss of LBM is due to abnormalities in micronutrient metabolism caused by alterations in regulatory hormones and cytokines, nutritional support may lead to body weight gain which is often the net result of increased fat deposition and increased body water, not an increase in LBM (Shike et al. 1984). LBM is more likely to be restored by nutritional therapy in patients with simple macronutrient deficiency than in those who have primary alterations in metabolism (Shike et al. 1984; Kotler et al. 1985; Klein et al. 1997).

A recent meta-analysis reported that aggressive nutritional support in surgical and critically ill patients who are known to be hypermetabolic (with a loss of 20–40 g/day of nitrogen) and have increased nutrient requirements, did not influence the overall mortality; however, it may reduce the complication rate in already undernourished patients (Heyland et al. 1998).

The timing of nutritional support in non-surgical patients and those who are critically ill is less clear, because of lack of evidence, but most previously well nourished minimally stressed patients will only require nutritional support if they are unable to eat for more than 10–14 days (Souba 1997).

12.2 Predictors of stroke patients' nutritional status during the hospital stay

A study conducted to explore possible prognostic nutritional and non-nutritional clinical indicators which may predict the serum albumin concentration as a measure of nutritional status during hospital stay in a cohort of acute stroke patients, and also to attempt to differentiate the effects of malnutrition from those of acute illness on the serum albumin concentration, found that most patients showed marked and significant deterioration in all measures of nutritional status during their hospital stay (Gariballa 2001). The increase in the amount of variance in serum albumin concentrations explained by nutritional variables between admission and week 4 is shown in Tables 12.1–12.3. The low average daily energy intake for both stroke patients and non-stroke patients without swallowing difficulties during the hospital stay is revealed in Table 12.4.

Amongst nutritional status assessment parameters, serum albumin is one of the most accurately measured and therefore offers the best hope. However, many conditions, such as catabolism associated with acute and sub acute illness, liver and renal disease, may reduce serum albumin concentrations. The catabolic state and the associated neuroendocrine response which is likely to follow an acute stroke may lead to altered serum albumin concentrations, and there is evidence linking the high stress reaction following stroke and hypoalbuminaemia (Davalos et al. 1996). It may therefore be that in catabolic states the synthesis of acute phase proteins has a priority over serum albumin, and this may partly account for some of the features of the plasma protein profile observed during the acute phase response after injury. It is also well known, however, that undernutrition negatively affects protein synthesis, and

Table 12.1 Multiple regression model to predict serum albumin on admission. Reproduced from Gariballa (2001) with permission of Elsevier Science.

Variable[a]	R square	Adjusted R square	R square change	Standard error of the estimate	P value
Age	0.087	0.081	0.087	3.55	0.000[b]
Previous illness	0.087	0.076	0.000	3.56	0.961
Drugs	0.89	0.072	0.002	3.57	0.530
Rankin score	0.119	0.098	0.031	3.52	0.017[b]
TSF	0.119	0.093	0.000	3.53	0.982
MAC	0.140	0.109	0.021	3.50	0.046[b]
Transferrin	0.190	0.155	0.050	3.40	0.002[b]
Serum iron	0.228	0.190	0.038	3.33	0.005[b]

[a] MAC, mid-arm circumference; TSF, triceps skin-fold thickness.
[b] $P < 0.05$.

Table 12.2 Multiple regression model to predict serum albumin at week 2. Reproduced from Gariballa (2001) with permission of Elsevier Science.

Variable[a]	R square	Adjusted R square	R square change	Standard error of the estimate	P value
Age	0.094	0.082	0.094	3.77	0.007[b]
Previous illness	0.138	0.115	0.044	3.70	0.056
Drugs	0.138	0.103	0.000	3.73	0.999
Rankin score	0.226	0.183	0.088	3.56	0.005[b]
TSF	0.228	0.174	0.002	3.58	0.694
MAC	0.289	0.228	0.061	3.46	0.017[b]
Transferrin	0.391	0.329	0.102	3.22	0.001[b]
Serum iron	0.436	0.370	0.045	3.12	0.022[b]

[a] For abbreviations, see Table 12.1.
[b] $P < 0.05$.

Table 12.3 Multiple regression model to predict serum albumin at week 4. Reproduced from Gariballa (2001) with permission of Elsevier Science.

Variable[a]	R square	Adjusted R square	R square change	Standard error of the estimate	P value
Age	0.044	0.019	0.044	3.58	0.193
Previous illness	0.158	0.112	0.114	3.41	0.032[b]
Drugs	0.187	0.120	0.030	3.39	0.260
Rankin score	0.297	0.216	0.109	3.20	0.026[b]
TSF	0.302	0.200	0.006	3.23	0.599
MAC	0.387	0.275	0.084	3.08	0.041[b]
Transferrin	0.538	0.437	0.151	2.71	0.003[b]
Serum iron	0.538	0.419	0.000	2.76	0.876

[a] For abbreviations, see Table 12.1
[b] $P < 0.05$.

Table 12.4 Comparison of predicted and in-hospital energy intakes between stroke patients and controls. Reproduced from Gariballa (2001) with permission of Elsevier Science.

	Predicted energy intake	Actual in-hospital energy intake	Mean difference	95% CI
Stroke	1808 (260)	1338 (390)	470[a,b]	239–701
Controls	1805 (359)	1317 (358)	488[b,c]	298–679

[a] $P = 0.001$.
[b] Between-group difference was not statistically significant.
[c] $P < 0.0001$.

it has been shown in man that nutrition is probably the single most important factor regulating albumin synthesis (Rothschild 1972a, b; Dionigi et al. 1986).

It has also been shown that low serum albumin levels were related to poor outcome, not just during the acute phase following the stroke, but also throughout the hospital stay, an effect unlikely to be explained by the catabolic state alone (Gariballa et al. 1998b,c). An attempt was made to control for a number of non-nutritional factors which were likely to affect outcomes, including several clinical indicators of stroke severity and level of co-morbidity, such as age, Rankin score, previous illnesses and the number of medications. Others (Agarwal 1988; Rich et al. 1989; Davalos et al. 1996) have also demonstrated a strong association between serum albumin levels and clinical outcome.

Other recent studies (Gariballa 2001; Gariballa et al. 1998b,c) seem to suggest that nutritional status as measured by serum albumin following acute stroke may be of more prognostic significance later on during the course of hospitalisation. This hypothesis is supported by the results of two studies of nutritional support of hospitalised acute stroke patients. In the first study (Davalos et al. 1996), nutritional support within the first week following the stroke did not prevent the decline in serum albumin concentrations. The latter study (Gariballa et al. 1998a), which was a randomised controlled single-blind trial, found that oral nutritional supplementation commencing 1 week following the stroke and continuing for a further 4 weeks during the hospital stay significantly improved nutritional intakes, prevented decline in serum albumin concentrations and had a favourable but non-significant impact on clinical outcome. The lack of statistical significance on clinical outcome was probably a reflection of the small sample size.

12.3   Nutritional status during rehabilitation and following discharge

The majority of stroke victims (> 75%) are elderly people who are more likely to have pre-morbid decrease in energy intake, less lean body mass and impaired immune response that may be associated with nutritional deficiencies (Morley 1986; Chandra 1997). Their nutritional status is likely to deteriorate further as the result of the catabolism associated with the acute illness (Klein et al. 1997). This is compounded further by the demands of the sometimes prolonged rehabilitation period. Two complementary studies of nutritional status and energy intake of 350 randomly selected admissions to a geriatric rehabilitation unit found that protein–energy undernutrition was a strong predictor of in-hospital and post-discharge mortality (Sullivan & Walls 1994; Sullivan et al. 1995). A recent study of predictors of early non-elective hospital re-admission in elderly patients has found that individuals with any amount of body weight loss and no improvement in albumin concentrations during the first month after hospitalisation were at a much higher risk of re-admission than were those who maintained or increased their post-discharge body weight and had repleted their serum albumin concentrations (Fried-mann et al. 1997).

Taken together, the results of above studies indicate that poor nutritional status following acute illness in ageing patients may be of prognostic significance and amenable to therapy later on during the convalescent phase.

12.4 Summary

Based on present evidence, it is possible that the poor outcome in elderly patients following acute illness may at least be partly due to undernutrition, and that aggressive nutritional support during the convalescent period is more likely to improve nutritional status and lead to better rehabilitation outcome, decreased readmission rate, improved quality of life and contribute to reducing health service costs. An important challenge in understanding the interactions between nutrition, ageing and disease is to determine the optimal timing and composition of nutritional therapy relative to a patient's metabolic stress, age and specific illness.

13 Nutritional Support of Elderly Stroke Patients

13.1 Introduction

Undernutrition is prevalent and often unrecognised in patients admitted to hospitals and institutions (Sandstrom et al. 1985; Elmstahl & Steen 1987). There is also evidence linking protein–energy undernutrition (PEU) or its markers with clinical outcomes in acute and non-acute care settings (Sullivan & Walls 1994; Sullivan et al. 1995; Gariballa et al. 1998a–c). Does nutritional supplementation improve nutritional intake, status and/or outcome of elderly stroke patients, and if so when would it be most effective? This chapter reviews recent research on nutritional support in hospitalised elderly stroke patients.

13.2 Why do elderly stroke patients need nutritional support?

Before coming into hospital, elderly people in the community are more likely to have pre-morbid decrease in energy intake, less lean body mass, and other related nutritional deficiencies (Morley 1986; Chandra 1997). Their nutritional status is likely to deteriorate further as the result of the catabolism associated with the acute illness, increased demands and reduced intake during the rehabilitation period (Davalos et al. 1996; Gariballa et al. 1998b,c).

A high proportion of stroke patients were found to have low anthropometric and biochemical values on admission and most patients remaining in hospital showed marked and significant deterioration in all measures of nutritional status during their stay (Gariballa et al. 1998b). After adjusting for poor prognostic indicators, nutritional status in hospital was found to be a strong and independent predictor of morbidity and mortality (Gariballa et al. 1998c).

13.3 Improving nutritional status in hospitalised elderly patients and its relation to clinical outcome

The only way to ascertain the benefit of nutritional supplements on undernourished elderly stroke patients is to carry out prospective randomised controlled intervention clinical trials. There have been positive results of trials

Table 13.1 Trials of nutritional intervention after acute stroke. From Gariballa (2000). Reproduced with permission from *British Journal of Nutrition*.

Authors & country	Participants	Comparison[a]	Sample size	Age (years)	Nutritional variables	Type and time of intervention	End-points[a]	Comments
Nyswonger & Helmchen 1992 USA	Retrospective review of records of stroke patients admitted to a community hospital who received enteral nutrition	Patients fed within 72 hours of admission (n = 20) compared with those fed later than 72 hours (n = 32)	52	(53–95)	According to assessment by the clinical dietician	Enteral nutrition within or later than 72 hours (not known for how long)	LOS	Significantly shorter LOS (SD) of 20.1 (12.9) days in those fed within 72 hours compared with those fed later than 72 hours LOS 29.8 (20.1) days
Norton et al. 1996 UK	Randomly selected stroke patients with persistent dysphagia and requiring enteral nutrition	PEG tube feeding (n = 16) versus NGT feeding (n = 14)	30 (11 males)	(mean) 77	Body weight, haemoglobin, albumin and MAC	PEG tube feeding compared with NGT 14 days after acute stroke using a standard enteral feed (Nutrison)	Percentage of prescribed feed received, nutritional status, LOS and mortality	Significant improvement in nutritional status and shorter LOS among PEG-tube fed patients compared with NGT grouop. Mortality also significantly lower in PEG-tube group (12%) compared with NGT group (57%). All PEG-tube fed group received prescribed feed compared with 78% of NGT group

Reference	Patients	Study design	n	Age	Measures	Intervention	Outcomes	Results
Davalos et al. 1996 Spain	Acute stroke patients within 24 hours of the stroke	Nutritional status before and after feeding	104 (67 males)	66 (10) (mean (SD))	TSF, MAC and serum albumin	Oral standard diet (2000 kcal and 16 g of nitrogen) or polymeric enteral nutrition (30 kcal/kg and 14 g of nitrogen) for dysphagic patients within 24 hours of admission	Nutritional status within 1 week of hospitalisation	Early enteral nutrition did not prevent malnutrition during first week of hospital stay
Gariballa et al. 1998a UK	Stroke patients with evidence of undernutrition and without swallowing difficulties within 1 week of the stroke	Patients were randomised to 4 weeks of oral nutritional supplements plus hospital food (n = 21) or hospital food alone (n = 21)	42 (19 males)	79 (9) (mean (SD))	Body weight, TSF, MAC, albumin, transferrin and iron	Hospital diet plus a twice daily oral nutritional supplement of ≥ 400 ml of Fortisip containing 600 kcal and 20 g of protein at 3:00 p.m. and 8:00 p.m. daily for 4 weeks or until death or discharge	Nutritional status, morbidity, LOS, discharge destination and mortality	Significant improvement in energy intake and nutritional status in the supplemented group compared with controls. Effect on clinical outcome among the supplemented group not statistically significant

a LOS, length of stay; NGT, nasogastric tube; PEG, percutaneous endoscopic gastrostomy.

of nutritional support given enterally or orally in comparable settings. Bastow et al. (1983) studied the effect of overnight nasogastric feeding supplements of 1000 kcal in a randomised controlled trial of elderly women with a fractured neck of femur and showed that treatment was associated with improvements, not only in anthropometric and plasma protein measurements, but also in clinical outcome, mainly in shortened rehabilitation time and hospital stay. Delmi et al. (1990) were able to demonstrate a clinical benefit of oral supplements in a randomised controlled group of elderly patients with fractured femur, which persisted 6 months after injury. In a randomised controlled trial Woo et al. (1994) demonstrated clinical benefit of oral supplements on a group of elderly patients suffering from chest infection. The powerful study of Larsson et al. (1990) on 501 elderly in-patients who were randomly allocated to receive oral supplements or ward meals only, demonstrated clear benefit of nutritional supplements in terms of mortality, hospital stay, mobility and probability of pressure sores. In a double-blind placebo-controlled trial (Chandra 1992), 96 independently living, healthy men and women over 65 years of age were randomly assigned to receive nutrient supplementation. Nutrient status and immunological variables were assessed at baseline and at 12 months, and the frequency of illness due to infection was ascertained. Subjects in the supplement group had higher numbers of certain-cells subsets and natural killer cells, enhanced proliferation response to mitogen, increased interleukin-2 production and higher antibody response. Supplementation with micronutrient significantly improved immunity and decreased the risk of infection. Another randomised placebo-controlled trial (Fiatarone et al. 1994), compared progressive resistance exercise training, multinutrient supplementation, both interventions and neither intervention in 100 frail nursing home residents over a 10-week period. High intensity resistance exercise was found to be a feasible and effective means of counteracting muscle weakness and physical frailty in very old people. In contrast, multinutrient supplementation without concomitant exercise did not reduce muscle weakness or physical frailty.

Some studies (Stableforth 1986; Williams et al. 1989; Hankey et al. 1993) have not shown a clear benefit of nutritional supplements on elderly hospital surgical and non-surgical patients; however, in these studies there were problems with compliance and tolerance of supplements, and almost all included smaller numbers of patients without adequate control for confounding variables compared with the studies that demonstrated a clear benefit.

13.4 Nutritional support following stroke

A review of the literature regarding early or late nutritional support following stroke did not reveal many studies in this area (Table 13.1). Despite methodological limitations, some studies have demonstrated that nutritional

Table 13.2 Nutritional status indices measured at week 0 and follow-up (weeks 2, 4 and 12) for supplemented group and controls. Reproduced from Gariballa et al. (1998a) with permission from the American Society for Parenteral and Enteral Nutrition.

Parameter[a]	Supplemented group						Control group					
	Week 0 (n = 21)		Follow-up (n = 18)		Mean change	95% CI	Week 0 (n = 21)		Follow-up (n = 13)		Mean change	95% CI
	Mean	SD	Mean	SD			Mean	SD	Mean	SD		
Body weight (kg)	57.3	9.2	57.5	9.0	0.2	−1.1–1.4	57.0	9.1	56.3	8.4	−0.7	−2.7–1.4
TSF (mm)	6.1	1.5	5.2	1.7	−0.9	−1.9–0.1	5.4	1.6	4.8	1.8	−0.6	−1.5–0.4
MAC (cm)	24.0	1.4	23.7	2.1	−0.3	−0.9–0.3	23.3	2.6	23.0	2.9	−0.3	−1.2–0.7
Albumin (range 35–55 g/l)	37.9	3.5	36.4	2.8	−1.5	−3.1–0.1[b]	39.4	4	34.9	4.7	−4.4	−6.6 to −2.3[b]
Transferrin (range 2–4 g/l)	3.0	0.7	3.1	0.7	0.1	−0.4–0.5	3.1	0.2	2.7	0.4	−0.3	−0.6–0.1
Iron (range 14–28 μmol/l)	10.2	4.7	12.8	8.7	2.6	−1.5–6.7[c]	13.5	6.5	10.8	6.1	−2.7	−5.6–0.2[c]

[a] MAC, mid-arm circumference; TSF, triceps skin-fold thickness. For the difference between the changes in the two groups.
[b] P = 0.025; 95% CI, −5.57 to −0.4).
[c] P = 0.030; 95% CI, −10.0 to −0.6).

Table 13.3 Secondary outcome measures for the supplements group compared with the controls. Reproduced from Gariballa et al. (1998a) with permission from the American Society for Parenteral and Enteral Nutrition.

	Supplemented group (*n* = 20)	Controls (*n* = 20)
Barthel score (week 0)[a]	45 (20–58.75)	35 (16.25–48.75)
Barthel score (follow-up)[a]	90 (60–93.75)	75 (47–87.5)
Length of stay (days)[a]	24 (3–122)	42 (3–77)
Number of infective complications	9	11
Death within 3 months	2	7
Discharge destination		
Own home	12	8
Relative's home	1	1
Residential home	2	1
Nursing home	3	3

[a] Median (inter-quartile range).

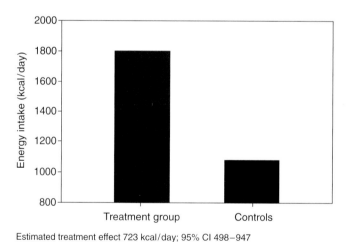

Estimated treatment effect 723 kcal/day; 95% CI 498–947

Figure 13.1 Mean energy intake of treatment group and controls.

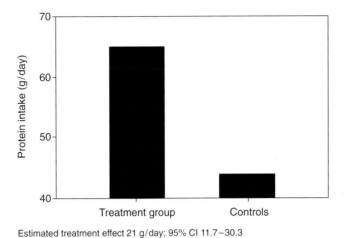

Estimated treatment effect 21 g/day; 95% CI 11.7–30.3

Figure 13.2   Mean protein intake of treatment group and controls.

support may have a positive role to play in the care and rehabilitation of patients with acute and chronic neurological problems including stroke patients (Gariballa & Sinclair 1998b). In one study, for example, nutritional support within 1 week of hospitalisation following stroke did not prevent undernutrition (Davalos et al. 1996). However, a randomised controlled single-blind trial (Gariballa et al. 1998a) showed that oral nutritional supplementation started 1 week after the stroke and continued for a further 4 weeks during the hospital stay significantly improved nutritional intakes, prevented decline in nutritional status and had a favourable but non-significant impact on clinical outcome (Tables 13.2, 13.3; Figures 13.1, 13.2). Thus, aggressive nutritional support during the convalescent period, rather than immediately following acute illness, is more likely to improve nutritional status and lead to better rehabilitation outcome, decreased readmission rate, improved quality of life, and contribute to reducing health service costs. Randomised controlled trials of nutritional support are therefore needed to determine the optimal timing and composition of nutritional therapy relative to a patient's metabolic stress and age. The ongoing FOOD trial, which is a multicentre randomised study evaluating various feeding policies after acute stroke, may help to answer some of the above questions.

13.5 Summary

There are now many studies which have found that undernutrition is prevalent and often unrecognised in stroke patients admitted to hospitals and institutions. There is also evidence which links protein–energy undernutrition or its markers with clinical outcomes in acute and non-acute stroke and non-stroke patients, and that nutritional supplements can improve outcomes in some of these settings. Active nutritional support following the catabolic phase of acute illness and extending through the rehabilitation period may be of particular benefit in improving nutritional intake, status and/or outcome.

14 Nutritional Status in the Community

14.1 Nutritional status of elderly people in the community

Risk factors for undernutrition amongst elderly people in the community include: isolation with an inability to go out shopping, loss of spouse, depression and bereavement, decreased mobility, dementia, anorexia due to disease (especially cancer), medications, poor dentition, alcoholism and, most important of all, acute illness. In institutions, lack of supervision and assistance at mealtimes may be an important factor resulting in poor food intake (Hoffman 1993).

There are conflicting viewpoints on the prevalence of undernutrition amongst elderly people in the community. Taylor (1980) in the UK and the Citizens' Board of Inquiry in the USA (1980) have implied that undernutrition is a widespread problem in the elderly. Taylor (1980) stated that classical signs of vitamin deficiency are found very commonly in elderly people in Great Britain and elsewhere. In contrast, both in Great Britain and in the USA, some studies found that undernutrition was an uncommon problem.

A detailed diet and nutrition survey was conducted in six towns in England and Scotland in 1967–1968, which used dietary recall and diary methods to assess energy and nutrient intakes. Full information was obtained from 764 people (Department of Health and Social Security 1972). There was a further study in 1972–1973 of 365 surviving elderly people who had participated in the 1967–1968 survey and who could be traced (Department of Health and Social Security 1979a). These surveys excluded people in institutional care. Among the findings in 1967–1968 were that 3% of those surveyed were diagnosed as being undernourished and three-quarters of these cases were in association with clinical disease. In 1972–1973 7% of the group surveyed were considered to be undernourished and this condition was more prevalent in those over 80 years of age. Several risk factors for undernutrition were identified of which the most important was being housebound. A major conclusion of this survey was that, provided individual elderly people were in good health, their dietary patterns and the foods eaten were no different from what is known about those of younger people. In 1986–1987, 2197 people aged 16 to 64 living in Great Britain recorded their weighed dietary intakes for 7 days, were measured for height, body weight and blood pressure, and provided blood and urine for analysis (Gregory et al. 1990); this survey provided information about the diet of a nationally representative sample of younger adults, and for reasons given above may reflect the dietary patterns of elderly people.

The studies in California by Morgan et al. (1955) showed that, although the intake of energy and nutrients fell with increasing age, when the results were expressed per unit body weight there was an insignificant decrease with ageing. The economic status of the population studied covered the entire spectrum and there were no signs of ageing which were affecting nutritional intake. Apart from a general reduction in all nutrients, there were few changes of nutritional significance in the same Californian population after 14 years follow-up. In the UK, results obtained by Lonergan et al. (1975) on energy intake of elderly men and women were similar to those of the Californian population. The study recorded dietary history covering 1 week for 212 men and 263 women aged 62–90 years living in Edinburgh. The histories were also validated by 2 days' weighed-diet records for 219 subjects. The mean energy intake was 2335 kcal per day for men and was 1700 kcal per day for women (Lonergan et al. 1975). In a study of 100 subjects receiving 'meals on wheels' in England, Davies and Holdsworth (1978) found that men between the ages of 65 and 74 years and those over the age of 75 years consumed almost identical quantities of energy: 2160 and 2150 kcal per day, respectively. However, women aged 65 to 74 years consumed 1600 kcal per day, whilst older women (over 75 years) unexpectedly consumed 1750 kcal per day. In a 10-year cohort comparison and a 6-year longitudinal prospective study of 70- and 76-year-old Swedish people from Gothenburg, Sjogren et al. (1994) studied the intake of energy, nutrients and food items. They found that intake of energy and almost all nutrients decreased in both men and women between the ages of 70 and 76 years; energy intake reduced by 23% in men and 20% in women. However, they concluded that there is no reason to believe elderly people are more conservative regarding their food choices than the rest of the population. In the Euronut SENECA Study, 2586 elderly subjects born between 1913 and 1918 were studied in 19 towns across Europe using a longitudinal mixed design (Euronut SENECA Investigators 1991). Data regarding nutrients and food intakes, dietary habits, diet awareness, nutritional status, health and lifestyle factors were collected. It was found that there was considerable variability from site to site, even within countries, both in quantity and composition of dietary intake, blood biochemistry, lifestyle factors, health and performance (de Groot et al. 1992). The average participation rate was 51% with wide variation among towns. Haemoglobin, haematocrit and serum albumin did not indicate that the 70–75-year-old subjects examined were in poor health. Considerable diversity and variability in serum lipid profile and dietary intakes of all components were observed. However, living conditions and social activities reflected a high quality of life and most of the elderly were still engaged in physical activities.

Because old people are disproportionately isolated, on low income or disabled, socioeconomic factors and disease are likely to have more influence on their nutritional status than age alone. As discussed in Chapter 2, a report from the USA showed an increase in disability with age from 3.5% of people aged 65–69 years who had difficulty preparing food rising to 26.1% of those aged over 85 years, whilst the numbers with difficulty shopping rose from 1.9% in the former group to 37% in the latter (Dawson et al. 1987). The Nottingham Longitudinal Survey of Activity and Ageing in the UK reported that 6% of women aged 65–74 years did not do their own cooking, rising to 12% of women aged over 74 years; 11% of women aged 65–74 years did not do their shopping, rising to 30% for those over 74 years (Dallosso 1988). Food associated problems and perceived health may also have a role to play. Ultimately, identification of those ambulatory elderly people at risk of undernutrition requires understanding of their social, cultural and economic environment.

Assessing nutritional status of individuals, especially elderly people living in the community, by cross-sectional and longitudinal surveys can be difficult, inaccurate and, at times, subject to major error. This may explain the conflicting results obtained by different researchers in the past. The cause for this may not just be differences in the methodologies of the various studies, but also biological factors related to the processes of ageing; for example, the representativeness of one sample selected for a study to the cohort of the elderly population at that time, and the inevitable march of mortality with time which reduces the numbers of a given cohort. Dietary habits of the cohort or the nation in general might have changed with times. Finally, the selective survival explanation assumes that those individuals who were better nourished at the start of a study will have outlived those who were initially less well nourished.

The most recent National Diet and Nutrition Survey (Finch et al. 1998) of British people aged 65 years and over found that the mean energy intake for free-living men was 1909 kcal and for women was 1422 kcal; 7% of men and 11% of women in the free-living group, and 13% of men and 12% of women in institutions reported that they had been unwell during the dietary recording period and their eating had been affected. In the free-living group, these participants were found to have, on average, lower intakes of protein, total carbohydrates and starch, although there was no significant difference in energy intake. Free-living men who were unwell and whose eating was affected had lower intakes of vitamins A, D, pantothenic acid and riboflavin, and lower intakes per unit of energy of retinol, vitamin B12 and vitamin D. These differences in vitamin intake were not seen in free-living women and there were few differences in institutions between those well and unwell.

14.2   Nutritional status of stroke patients in the community

The majority of stroke victims are elderly people, and stroke is the most important single cause of severe disability among Western people living in their own homes; therefore, the prevalence of nutritional disorders amongst stroke victims living in the community is likely to be very high. However, there is little knowledge available about the types and extent of nutritional disorders and their relationship to the health and well-being of community stroke residents. Westergren et al. (2001) studied the types and extent of eating difficulties, the need for assistance when eating, the nutritional status and pressure ulcers of 162 consecutive stroke patients admitted for rehabilitation over a period of 1 year. Out of 162 patients 80% were found to have had eating difficulties, whilst 52.5% were dependent on assisted eating. Eating difficulties were, in decreasing order: 'eats three-quarters or less of served food', difficulties in 'manipulating food on the plate', in 'transportation of food to the mouth', in the 'sitting position', 'aberrant eating speed', 'manipulating food in the mouth', 'swallowing difficulties', 'opening and/or closing the mouth' and 'alertness'. The patient's situation before stroke and the effects of the stroke influenced the need for assisted eating. When admitted for stroke rehabilitation, 32% were at risk of or were already undernourished, this being significantly more common among patients needing assisted eating than among those with no such need. The conclusion of this study was that eating difficulties among patients with stroke were characterised by great complexity, and exist among both patients who need assisted eating and those who do not. The most common eating difficulties were those related to the phase before the food reaches the mouth. Some eating difficulties showed significant predictive ability for undernourishment, which in turn increased the likelihood of also having pressure ulcers.

A study from the Republic of Ireland examining the state of patients on enteral tube feeding in the community found that 46% of patients required such feeding as a consequence of swallowing difficulties caused by stroke compared with 24% of patients who needed enteral tube feeding because of swallowing difficulties caused by cancer. Stroke patients were found to have poor functional ability and nutritional assessment proved difficult to carry out on many of them. Problems encountered with feeding included blocked tubes (30%), infected stoma sites (16%), and logistical problems regarding feed and equipment. Nutritional follow-up was not routine in patients with poor mobility, and 55% of patients on long-term tube feeding had not been reviewed by a dietitian in over 1 year (McNamara et al. 2000). A complementary paper assessing the contribution of health professionals to the care of patients on enteral tube feeding in the community found that hospital dietitians carry out most of the initial education and training of patients, in addition to the nutritional aftercare. General practitioners tend not to be involved, and there is a need to improve co-ordination between hospital and community services; more consistent monitoring of those on home enteral tube feeding would be advantageous for such patients (McNamara et al. 2001).

14.3 Summary

Several factors operate together to produce undernutrition in certain sections of elderly people living in the community, including stroke patients. For example, limited mobility, loneliness, social isolation, difficulties in swallowing, physical and mental frailty, are all common in housebound old people. Undernutrition can adversely affect physical, psychological and behavioural function, and this can have major social and economic implications. The extent and impact of nutritional disorders on community stroke patients is not fully understood and needs further research.

15 Future Directions and Recommendations

15.1 Areas for further research

Observational studies have demonstrated that dietary factors may have an important role to play in incidence, clinical course and outcome of stroke; however, causal association is not definitely established. Therefore, there is an urgent need for further research in certain areas such as:

(1) Environmental factors, including diet, may be important in the genesis of stroke and in the potential to prevent its occurrence. At present, most of the evidence in humans is observational and therefore does not establish causal relationship. Large-scale experimental studies are needed to provide compelling data on which sound and scientific dietary advice to patients could be based.

(2) There is growing support for the involvement of free radicals and other micronutrients in atherosclerotic diseases, e.g. stroke and ischaemic heart disease, all of which may be associated with nutritional problems. If so, the therapeutic rewards may be great. There is a need to develop and validate better techniques for direct measurements of antioxidant capacity and oxidative stress, and adjust for confounding variables.

(3) The protective effects of intake of fruits and vegetables may not wholly be attributable to their antioxidant content. Other currently unmeasured essential nutrients may have equal protective properties. This area is in need of basic research.

(4) The use of antioxidants for the treatment of human cardiovascular diseases has produced contradictory results. The explanation for this paradox may be that antioxidants can give protective effects or worsen damage depending on the timing of administration in relation to the sequence of events (ischaemia and reperfusion in the case of myocardial infarction and ischaemic stroke). As Halliwell (2000) stated, 'We do not administer antihypertensive drugs to patients in clinical trials without checking blood pressure, so why should we give antioxidants without checking that they have decreased oxidant status?'

(5) Energy requirements and expenditure after acute stroke and particularly during rehabilitation are of particular interest. Techniques to measure

energy requirements and expenditure in these patients need to be validated.

(6) There is some evidence that nutritional support during convalescence may improve nutritional status in hospital and thereafter in the community. A randomised controlled trial of nutritional support to determine the optimal timing and composition of nutritional therapy relative to a patient's metabolic stress and age is needed to test this hypothesis.

(7) At present it is not known how much poor nutrient intake contributes to the poor outcome which often follows PEG-tube insertion, and whether improving the nutritional status before PEG-tube insertion would influence the outcome. This important area is in need of urgent research.

(8) Despite aggressive nutritional support, it is often difficult to attenuate the catabolic response to illness or injury. Several new strategies to achieve this are under investigation. These include the administration of growth hormone to promote anabolism, essential amino acids such as glutamine, and nutrients that can modulate immune function. Although the use of these agents has been advocated, their benefits remain controversial and further studies are needed to establish their efficacy.

15.2   Recommendations on dietary and nutritional factors

15.2.1   Primary and secondary prevention of stroke

(1) Maintain diet that is rich in fruits and vegetables (at least five servings per day), legumes, fish, grains and cereals. For folate, as well as vitamins B6 and B12 replace deficiencies when identified. Emphasis should also be placed on meeting current RDAs. In high-risk patients, screening for fasting plasma homocysteine may be justified.

(2) Maintain energy balance and ideal body weight through diet and regular exercise.

(3) Limit excess intake of saturated fat, sodium and alcohol.

15.2.2   Strokes in hospital and the community

(1) Dietetic advice must be regarded as an integral part of the management of stroke patients in hospital. It should be sought early to assess the most appropriate method of meeting individual nutritional requirements in those stroke patients at risk, and provide advice for nursing and medical staff, catering and other health professionals involved.

(2) Assessment of nutritional status should be a routine aspect of history

taking and clinical examination when a stroke patient is admitted to hospital.

(3) Stroke patients at risk of undernutrition on admission include those with prior evidence of undernutrition, those who lived alone or in an institution before admission, or those with swallowing difficulties and/or incontinence of urine.

(4) A serum albumin concentration is a simple biochemical index of nutritional status and should be measured early after admission and periodically during the hospital stay.

(5) Assistance should be provided to stroke patients to make the right food choices, and to feed them if necessary.

(6) Priorities should be given to mealtimes; nursing supervision should be available and stroke patients should be allowed enough time to eat.

(7) Doctors, nurses and members of the multidisciplinary team looking after stroke patients should be made aware of the impact of nutritional status on stroke outcome.

(8) When recommending PEG-tube feeding to a dysphagic stroke patient, the treating doctor has a duty to undertake adequate consultation with competent patients, closest relatives and all members of the multidisciplinary team involved with the patient before recommending the procedure.

References

Abbott, R.D., Behrens, G.R., Sharp, D.S., Rodriguez, B.L., Burchfiel, C.M., Ross, G.W., Yano, K. & Curb, J.D. (1994). Body mass index and thromboembolic stroke. *Stroke* **25**, 2370–2376.

Abbott, R.D., Curb, J.D., Rodriguez, B.L., Sharp, D.S., Burchfiel, C.M. & Yano, K. (1996). Effect of dietary calcium and milk consumption on risk of thromboembolic stroke in older middle-aged men. *Stroke* **27**, 813–818.

Abe, Y., El-Masri, B., Kimball, K.T., Pownall, H., Reilly, C.F., Osmundsen, K., Smith, C.W. & Ballantyne, C.M. (1998). Soluble cell adhesion molecules in hypertriglyceridemia and potential significance on monocyte adhesion. *Arterioscler. Thromb. Vasc. Biol.* **18**, 723–731.

Acheson, R.M. & Williams, D.R.R. (1983). Does consumption of fruit and vegetables protect against stroke? *Lancet* **28**, 1191–1193.

Adams, M.R., McCredie, R., Jessup, W., Robinson, J., Sullivan, D. & Celermajer, D.S. (1997). Oral L-arginine improves endothelium-dependent dilatation and reduces monocyte adhesion to endothelial cells in young men with coronary artery disease. *Atherosclerosis* **129**, 261–269.

Agarwal, N., Acevedo, F., Leighton, L., Cayten, C.G. & Pitchumoni, C.S. (1988). Predictive ability of various nutritional variables for mortality in elderly people. *Am. J. Clin. Nutr.* **48**, 1173–1178.

Albertini, J.P., Valensi, P., Lormeau, B., Aurousseau, M.H., Ferriere, F., Attali, J.R. & Gattengno, L. (1998). Elevated concentrations of soluble E-selectin and vascular cell adhesion molecule-1 in NIDDM. Effects of intensive insulin treatment. *Diabetes Care* **21**, 1008–1013.

Alfthan, G., Pekkanen, J., Jauhiainen, M., Pitkaniemi, J., Karvonen, M., Tuomilehto, J., Salonen, J.T. & Ehnholm, C. (1994). Relation of serum homocysteine and lipoprotein (a) concentrations to atherosclerotic disease in a prospective Finnish population based study. *Atherosclerosis* **106**, 9–19.

Alpha-Tocopherol, Beta Carotene Cancer Prevention Study Group (1994). The effect of vitamin E and beta carotene on the incidence of lung cancer and other cancers in male smokers. *New Engl. J. Med.* **330**, 1029–1035.

Altura, B.T., Burton, M. & Altura, M. (1984). Interactions of Mg and K on cerebral vessels – aspects in view of stroke. *Magnesium* **3**, 195–211.

Aminbakhsh, A. & Mancini, J. (1999). Chronic antioxidant use and changes in endothelial dysfunction: a review of clinical investigations. *Can. J. Cardiol.* **15**, 895–903.

Andersson, T.L., Matz, J., Ferns, G.A. & Anggard, E.E. (1994). Vitamin E reverses cholesterol-induced endothelial dysfunction in the rabbit coronary circulation. *Atherosclerosis* **111**, 39–45.

Aptaker, R.L., Roth, E.J., Reichhardt, G., Querden, M.E. & Levy, C.E. (1994). Serum albumin level as a predictor of geriatric stroke rehabilitation outcome. *Arch. Phys. Med. Rehabil.* **75**, 80–84.

Armstead, W.M., Mirro, R., Busija, C.W. & Leffler, C.W. (1988). Postischaemic generation of superoxide anion by newborn pig brain. *Am. J. Physiol.* **255**(24), H401–H403.

Arnesen, E., Refsum, H., Bonaa, K.J., Ueland, P.M., Forde, O.H. & Nordrehaug, J.E. (1995). Serum total homocysteine and coronary heart disease. *Int. J. Epidemiol.* **24**, 704–709.

Ascherio, A., Rimm, E.B., Hernan, M.A., Giovannucci, E.L., Kawachi, I., Stampfer, M.J. & Willett, W.C. (1998). Intake of potassium, magnesium, calcium and fiber and risk of stroke among US men. *Circulation* **98**, 1198–1204.

Axelsson, K., Norberg, A. & Asplund, K. (1984). Eating after stroke. *Intl Nurs. Stud.* **21**(2), 93–99.

Axelsson, K., Asplund, K., Norberg, A. & Alafuzoff, I. (1988). Nutritional status in patients with acute stroke. *Acta Med. Scand.* **224**, 217–224.

Axelsson, K., Asplund, K., Norberg, A. & Eriksson, S. (1989). Eating problems of patients with severe stroke. *J. Am. Dietet. Assoc.* **89**, 1092–1096.

Bajorunas, D.R. (1999). Micronutrients in cardiovascular nutrition: rationale and dosing considerations. *Heart Failure* **15**, 165–178.

Bamford, J., Sandercock, P., Dennis, M., Warlow, C., Jones, L., McPherson, K., Vessey, M., Fowler, G., Molyneux, A., Hughes, T., Burn, J. & Wade, D. (1988). A prospective study of acute cerebrovascular disease in the community. *J. Neurol. Neurosurg. Psychiatry* **61**, 1373–1380.

Bannan, S., Mansfield, M.W. & Grant, P.J. (1998). Soluble vascular cell adhesion molecule-1 and E-selectin levels in relation to vascular risk factors and to E-selectin genotype in the first degree relatives of NIDDM patients and NIDDM patients. *Diabetologia* **41**, 460–466.

Barer, D., Leibowitz, R., Ebrahim, S., Pengally, D. & Neale, R. (1989). Vitamin C status in patients with stroke and other acute illnesses. *J. Clin. Epidemiol.* **42**(7), 625–631.

Barker, D.J. (1997). Foetal nutrition and cardiovascular disease in later life. *Br. Med. Bull.* **53**, 96–108.

Barker, D.J.P., Osmond, C. & Pannett, B. (1992). Why Londoners have low death rates from ischaemic heart disease and stroke. *Br. Med. J.* **305**, 1551–1554.

Bassey, E.J. (1986). Demispan as a measure of skeletal size. *Ann. Hum. Biol.* **13**, 499–502.

Bassey, E.J. & Harries, U.J. (1993). Normal values for handgrip strength in 920 men and women aged over 65 years, and longitudinal changes over 4 years in 620 survivors. *Clin. Sci.* **84**(3), 331–337.

Bassey, E.J. & Terry, A.M. (1986). The oxygen cost of walking in the elderly. *J. Physiol* **373**, 42 (abstract).

Bassey, E.J. & Terry, A.M. (1988). Blood lactate in relation to oxygen uptake during uphill treadmill walking in young and old women. *J. Physiol.* **396**, 104 (abstract).

Bastow, M.D., Rawlings, J. & Allison, S.P. (1983). Benefits of supplementary tube feeding after fractured neck of femur. *Br. Med. J.* **287**, 1589–1592.

Bath, P.M.W., Bath, F.J. & Smithard, D.G. (2002). Interventions for dysphagia in acute stroke. The Cochrane Library, Issue 4. John Wiley & Sons, Chichester.

Baumgartner, R.N. (1995). Body weight and weight changes in elderly persons. *Facts Res. Gerontol.* **3**, 7–15.

Beamer, N., Coull, B.M., Sexton, G., de Garmo, P., Knox, R. & Seaman, G. (1993). Fibrinogen and the albumin–globulin ratio in recurrent stroke. *Stroke* **24**, 1133–1139.

Beaumont, D., Lehmann, A.B. & James, O.F.W. (1989). Protein turnover in malnourished elderly subjects: the effect of refeeding. *Age Ageing* **18**, 235–240.

Becker, B.F. (1993). Towards the physiological function of uric acid. *Free Radicals Biol. Med.* **14**, 615–631.

Beckman, J.S., Beckman, T.W., Chen, J., Marshall, P.A. & Freeman, B.A. (1990). Apparent hydroxyl radical production by peroxynitrite: implications for endothelial injury from nitric oxide and superoxide. *Proc. Natl Acad. Sci. USA* **87**, 1620–1624.

Bellamy, M.F., McDowell, I.F., Ramsey, M.W., Brownlee, M., Bones, C., Newcombe, R.G. & Lewis, M.J. (1998a). Hyperhomocysteinemia after an oral methionine load acutely impairs endothelial function in healthy adults. *Circulation* **98**, 1848–1852.

Bellamy, M.F., Goodfellow, J., Tweddel, A.C., Dunstan, F.D., Lewis, M.J. & Henderson, A.H. (1998b). Syndrome X and endothelial dysfunction. *Cardiovasc. Res* **40**, 410–417.

Bellamy, M.F., McDowell, I.F., Ramsey, M.W., Brownlee, M., Newcombe, R.G. & Lewis, M.J. (1999). Oral folate enhances endothelial function in hyperhomocysteinaemic subjects. *Eur. J. Clin. Invest.* **29**, 659–662.

Bergmann, S., Siekmeier, R., Mix, C. & Jaross, W. (1998). Even moderate cigarette smoking influences the pattern of circulating monocytes and concentration of sICAM-1. *Respir. Physiol.* **114**, 269–275.

Bertron, P., Barnard, N.D. & Mills, M. (1999). Racial bias in federal nutrition policy, Part II: Weak guidelines take a disproportionate toll. *J. Natl Med. Assoc.* **91**, 201–208.

Betz, A.L. (1985). Identification of hypoxanthine transport and xanthine oxidase activity in brain capillaries. *J. Neurochem.* **44**, 574–579.

Bhanthumnavin, K. & Schuster, M.D. (1977). In *Handbook of the Biology of Ageing* (Finch, C. & Hayflick, L. eds), p. 709. Van Nostrand Reinhold, New York.

Biller, J., Feinberg, W.M., Castaldo, J.E., Whittemore, A.D., Harbaugh, R.E., Dempsey, R.J., Caplan, L.R., Kresowik, T.F., Matchar, D.B., Toole, J.F. et al. (1998). Guidelines for carotid endarterectomy: a statement for healthcare professionals, American Heart Association. *Circulation* **97**, 501–509.

Bingham, S.A. (1987). The dietary assessment of individuals: methods, accuracy, new techniques and recommendations. *Nut. Abstr. Rev.* (Ser. A) **57**(10), 707–742.

Blair, S.N., Kampert, J.B., Kohl, H.W., Barlow, C.E., Marera, C.A., Paffenbarger, R.S. Jr & Gibbons, L.W. (1996). Influences of cardiorespiratory fitness and other precursors on cardiovascular disease and all-cause mortality in men and women. *J. Am. Med. Assoc.* **276**, 205–210.

Blann, A.D., Steele, C. & McCollum, C.N. (1997). The influence of smoking on soluble adhesion molecules and endothelial cell markers. *Thromb. Res.* **85**, 433–438.

Blum, A., Porat, R., Rosenschein, U., Keren, G., Roth, A., Laniado, S. & Miller, H. (1999). Clinical and inflammatory effects of dietary L-arginine in patients with intractable angina pectoris. *Am. J. Cardiol.* **83**, 1488–1490.

Blum, A., Hathaway, L., Mincemoyer, R., Schenke, W.H., Kirby, M., Csako, G., Wacl-wiw, M.A., Panza, J.A. & Cannon, R.O. (2000a). Oral L-arginine in patients with coronary artery disease on medical management. *Circulation* **101**, 2160–2164.

Blum, A., Hathaway, L., Mincemoyer, R., Schenke, W.H., Kirby, M., Csako, G., Waclawiw, M.A., Panza, J.A. & Cannon, R.O. (2000b). Effects of oral L-arginine on endothelium-dependent vasodilation and markers of inflammation in healthy post-menopausal women. *J. Am. Coll. Cardiol.* **35**, 271–276.

Bogden, J.D., Oleske, J.M., Lavenhar, M.A., Munves, E.M., Kemp, F.W., Blruening, K.S. Holding, K.J., Denny, T.N., Guarino, M.A., Krieger, L.M. & Holland, B.K. (1988). Zinc and immunocompetence in elderly people: effect of zinc supplementation for 3 months *Am. J. Clin. Nutri.* **8**, 655–663.

Bonita, R. Epidemiology of stroke (1992). *Lancet* **339**, 342–344.

Bostom, A.G. & Lathrop P.L. (1997). Homocysteinemia in end-stage renal disease: prevalence, etiology, and potential relationship to arteriosclerotic outcomes. *Kidney Int.* **52**, 10–20.

Boushey, C.J., Beresford, S.A.A., Omenn, G.S. & Motulsky, A.G. (1995). A quantitative assessment of plasma homocysteine as a risk factor for vascular disease: probable benefits of increasing folic acid intake. *J. Am. Med. Assoc.* **274**, 1049–1057.

Brattstrom, L. & Wilcken, D.E.L. (2000). Homocysteine and cardiovascular disease: cause or effect? *Am. J. Clin. Nutr.* **72**, 315–323.

Brattstrom, L., Lindgren, A., Israelsson, B., Malinow, M.R., Norrving, B., Upson, B. & Hamfelt, A. (1992). Hyperhomocysteinaemia in stroke: prevalence, cause and relationships to type of stroke and stroke risk factors. *Eur. J. Clin. Invest.* **22**, 214–221.

Brittain, K.R., Peet, S.M. & Castleden, C.M. (1998). Stroke and incontinence. *Stroke* **29**, 524–528.

Brocklehurst, J.C., Griffiths, L.L., Taylor, G.F., Marks, J., Scott, D.L. & Blackley, J. (1968). The clinical features of chronic vitamin deficiency – a therapeutic trial in geriatric hospital patients. *Gerontol. Clin.* **10**, 309–320.

Brown, A.A. & Hu, F.B. (2001). Dietary modulation of endothelial function: implications for cardiovascular disease. *Am. J. Clin. Nutr.* **73**(4), 673–686.

Buelow, J.M. & Jamieson, D. (1990). Potential for altered nutritional status in stroke patients. *Rehabil. Nurs.* **15**(5), 260 (abstract).

Bunker, V.W. & Clayton, B.E. (1989). Studies in the nutrition of elderly people with particular reference to essential trace elements. *Age Ageing* **18**, 422–429.

Burr, M.L. & Philips, K.M. (1984). Anthropometric norms in the elderly. *Br. J. Nutr.* **51**, 165–169.

Busse, E.W. (1980). Eating in late life: physiological and psychological factors. *Am. Pharmacol.* **20**(5), 36–38.

Buzby, G.P., Mullen, J.I., Mathews, D.C., Hobbs, C.L. & Rosato, E.F. (1979). Prognostic nutritional index in gastrointestinal surgery. *Am. J. Surg.* **139**, 160–167.

Campbell, W.W., Crim, M.C., Dallal, G.E., Young, V.R. & Evans, W.J. (1994). Increased protein requirements in elderly people. *Am. J. Clin. Nutr.* **60**, 501–509.

Cao, W., Carney, J.M., Duchon, A., Floyd, R.A. & Chevion, M. (1988). Oxygen radical involvement in ischaemia and reperfusion injury to brain. *Neurosci. Lett.* **88**, 233–238.

Ceballos-Picot, I., Merad-Boudia, M., Nicole, A., Thevenin, M., Hellier, G., Legrain, S. & Berr, C. (1996). Peripheral antioxidant enzyme activities and selenium in elderly subjects. *Free Radicals Biol. Med.* **20**, 579–587.

Ceriello, A., Falletti, E., Taboga, C., Tonutti, L., Ezsol, Z., Gonano, F. & Bartoli, E. (1998). Hyperglycemia-induced circulating ICAM-1 increase in diabetes mellitus: the possible role of oxidative stress. *Horm. Metab. Res.* **30**, 146–149.

Chambers, J.C., McGregor, A., Jean-Marie, J., Obeid, O.A. & Kooner, J.S. (1999a).

Demonstration of rapid onset vascular endothelial dysfunction after hyperhomocysteinemia: an effect reversible with vitamin C therapy. *Circulation* **99**, 1156–1160.

Chambers, J.C., Obeid, O.A. & Kooner, J.S. (1999b). Physiological increments in plasma homocysteine induce vascular endothelial dysfunction in normal human subjects. *Arterioscler. Thromb.* **19**, 2922–2927.

Chan, P.H. & Fishman, R.A. (1980). Transient formation of superoxide radicals in polyunsaturated fatty acid-induced brain swelling. *J. Neurochem.* **35**, 1004–1007.

Chan, P.H. & Fishman, R.A. (1987). Brain oedema: induction in cortical slides by polyunsaturated fatty acids. *Science* **201**, 358–360.

Chan, P.H., Kerlan, R. & Fishman, R.A. (1983). Reduction of γ-aminobutyric acid and glutamate uptake and (Na + K)-ATPase activity in brain slices and synaptosomes by arachidonic acid. *J. Neurochem.* **40**, 309–316.

Chandra, R.K. (1983). Nutrition, immunity and infection: present knowledge and future directions. *Lancet* **1**, 688–691.

Chandra, R.K. (1989). Nutritional regulation of immunocompetence and risk of disease. In: *Nutrition in the Elderly* (Horwitz, A., MacFadyen, D.M., Munro, H., Scrimshaw, N.S., Steen, B. & Williams, T.F., eds), pp. 203–218. Oxford University Press, Oxford.

Chandra, R.K. (1992). Effect of vitamin and trace-element supplementation on immune response and infection in elderly people. *Lancet* **340**, 1124–1127.

Chandra, R.K. (1997). Nutrition and the immune system: an introduction. *Am. J. Clin. Nutr.* **66**, 460S–463S.

Chang, H.R. & Bistrian, B. (1997). The role of cytokines in the catabolic consequences of infection and injury. *J. Parent. Ent. Nutr.* **22**, 156–166.

Chasan-Taber, L., Selhub, J., Rosenberg, I.H., Malinow, M.R., Terry, P., Tishler, P.V., Willet, W., Hennekens, C.H. & Stampfer, M.J. (1996). A prospective study of folate and vitamin B6 and risk of myocardial infarction in US physicians. *J. Am. Coll. Nutr.* **15**, 136–143.

Chee, D. & Stamler, J. (1999). Dietary folate and risk of cardiovascular mortality: results from the Multiple Risk Factor Intervention Trial (MRFIT). *Circulation* **100**(18), 4589 (Suppl.).

Cherubini, A., Polidori, M.C., Bregnocchi, M., Pezzuto, S., Cecchetti, R., Ingegni, T., de Iorio, A., Senin, U. & Mecocci, P. (2000). Antioxidant profile and early outcome in stroke patients. *Stroke* **31**, 2295–2300.

Choi-Kwon, S., Yang, Y.H., Kim, E.K., Jeon, M.Y. & Kim, J.S. (1998). Nutrition status in acute stroke: undernutrition versus overnutrition on different stroke subtypes. *Acta Neurol. Scand.* **98**, 187–192.

Christou, N.V., Meakins, J.L., Gordon, J., Yee, J., Hassan, Z.M., Nohr, C.W., Shizgal, H.M. & MacLean, L.D. (1995). The delayed hypersensitivity response and host resistance in surgical patients: 20 years later. *Ann. Surg.* **222**, 534–548.

Chumlea, W.C., Baumgartner, R.N., Garry, P.J., Rhyne, R.L., Nickolson, C & Wayne, S. (1992). Fat distribution and blood lipids in a sample of healthy elderly people. *Int. J. Obesity* **16**, 125–133.

Cino, M. & Del Maestro, R.F. (1989). Generation of hydrogen peroxide by brain mitochondria: the effect of reoxygenation following decapitative ischaemia. *Arch. Biochem. Biophys.* **269**, 623–638.

Citizens' Board of Inquiry into Hunger and Malnutrition in the United States (1980).

Hunger USA, pp. 1–100. Citizens' Crusade Against Poverty (Chairman, W.P. Reuther), Washington DC.

Clark, W.M., Lauten, J.D., Lessov, N., Woodward, W. & Coull, B.M. (1995). Time course of ICAM-1 expression and leucocyte subset infiltration in rat forebrain ischaemia. *Mol. Chem. Neuropath.* **26**, 213–230.

Clarke, R., Daly, L., Robinson, K., Naughten, E., Cahalane, S., Fowler, B. & Graham, I. (1991). Hyperhomocysteinemia: an independent risk factor for vascular disease. *New Engl. J. Med.* **324**, 1149–1155.

Clarkson, P., Adams, M.R., Powe, A.J., Donald, A.E., McCredie, R., Robinson, J., McCarthy, S.N., Keech, A., Celermajer, D.S. & Deanfield, J.E. (1996). Oral L-arginine improves endothelium-dependent dilation in hypercholesterolemic young adults. *J. Clin. Invest.* **97**, 1989–1994.

Cockerill, G.W., Rye, K.A., Gamble, J.R., Vadas, M.A. & Barter, P.J. (1995). High-density lipoproteins inhibit cytokine-induced expression of endothelial cell adhesion molecules. *Arterioscler. Thromb. Vasc. Biol.* **15**, 1987–1994.

Coles, J.C., Ahmed, S.N., Mehta, H.U. & Kaufman, J.C.E. (1986). Role of radical scavenger in protection of spinal cord during ischaemia. *Ann. Thorac. Surg.* **41**, 551–556.

Constans, J., Blann, A.D., Resplandy, F., Parrot, F., Renard, M., Seigneur, M., Guerin, V., Boisseau, M. & Conri, C. (1999). Three months' supplementation of hyperhomocysteinaemic patients with folic acid and vitamin B6 improves biological markers of endothelial dysfunction. *Br. J. Haematol.* **107**, 776–778.

Cooke, J.P. (2000). The endothelium: a new target for therapy. *Vasc. Med.* **5**, 49–53.

Cooper, A.J.L., Pulsinelli, W.A. & Duffy, T.E. (1980). Glutathione and ascorbate during ischaemia and postischaemic reperfusion in rat brain. *J. Neurochem.* **35**, 1242–1245.

Crouse, P.R., Byington, R.P., Hoen, H.M. & Furberg, C.D. (1997). Reductase inhibitor monotherapy and stroke prevention. *Arch. Int. Med.* **157**, 1305–1310.

Dallosso, H.M., Morgan, K., Bassey, E.J., Ebrahim, S.B., Fentem, P.H. & Arie, T.H. (1988). Levels of customary physical activity among the old and the very old living at home. *J. Epidemiol. Community Health* **42**, 121–127.

Davalos, A., Ricart, W., Gonzalez-Huix, F., Soler, S., Marrugat, J., Molins, A., Suner, R. & Genis, D. (1996). Effect of malnutrition after acute stroke on clinical outcome. *Stroke* **27**, 1028–1032.

Davi, G., Romano, M., Mezzetti, A., Procopio, A., Iacobelli, S., Antidormi, T., Bucciarelli, T., Alessandrini, P., Cuccurullo, F. & Bittolo Bon, G. (1998). Increased levels of soluble P-selectin in hypercholesterolemic patients. *Circulation* **97**, 953–957.

Davies, L. & Holdsworth, M.D. (1978). The place of milk in the diet of the elderly. *J. Hum. Nutr.* **32**, 195–200.

Davies, M.J. (1995). Stability and instability: two faces of coronary atherosclerosis. The Paul Dudley White Lecture. *Circulation* **94**, 2013–2020.

Dawson, D., Hendershot, G. & Fulton, J. (1987). Ageing in the eighties: functional limitations of individuals 65 and over. *NCHS Advance Data from Vital Health Statistics no. 133*, DHHS publication (PHS) 87-1250. Public Health Service, Hyattsville.

Dawson-Hughes, B., Harris, S.S., Krall, E.A. & Dallal, G.E. (1997). Effect of calcium and vitamin D supplementation on bone density in men and women 65 years of age and older. *New Engl. J. Med.* **337**, 670–676.

De Bono, D.P. (1994). Free radicals and antioxidants in vascular biology: the role of reaction kinetics, environment and substrate turnover. *Q. J. Med.* **87**, 445–453.

De Caterina, R., Cybulsky, M.I., Clinton, S.K., Gimbrone, M.A. & Libby, P. (1994). The omega-3 fatty acid docosahexaenoate reduces cytokine-induced expression of pro-atherogenic and proinflammatory proteins in human endothelial cells. *Arterioscler. Thromb.* **14**, 1829–1836.

De Caterina, R., Bernini, W., Carluccio, M.A., Liao, J.K. & Libby, P. (1998). Structural requirements for inhibition of cytokine-induced endothelial activation by unsaturated fatty acids. *J. Lipid Res.* **39**, 1062–1070.

De Caterina, R., Liao, J.K. & Libby, P. (2000). Fatty acid modulation of endothelial activation. *Am. J. Clin. Nutr.* **71**(suppl), 213S–23S.

DeGraba, T. (1998). The role of inflammation after stroke: utility of pursuing anti-adhesion molecule therapy. *Neurology* **51**(3), 62–68.

DeGraba, T.J., Siren, A.L., Penix, L., McCarron, R.M., Hargraves, R., Sood, S., Pettigrew, K.D. & Hallenbeck, J.M. (1998). Increased endothelial expression of intercellular adhesion molecule-1 in symptomatic versus asymptomatic human carotid athero-sclerosic plaque. *Stroke* **29**(7),1405–1410.

de Groot, L., Hautvast, J. & Staveren, W. (1992). Nutrition and health of elderly people in Europe: The Euronut–SENECA Study. *Nutr. Rev.* **50**(7), 185–194.

De Jong, S.C., Stehouwer, C.D., van den Berg, M., Geurts, T.W., Bouter, L.M. & Rauwerda, J.A. (1999). Normohomocysteinaemia and vitamin-treated hyperhomo-cysteinaemia are associated with similar risks of cardiovascular events in patients with premature peripheral arterial occlusive disease. A prospective cohort study. *J. Int. Med.* **1246**, 87–96.

De Keyser, J., De Klippel, N., Merkx, H., Vervaeck, M. & Merroelen, L. (1992). Serum concentrations of vitamin A and E and early outcome after ischaemic stroke. *Lancet* **339**, 1562–1565.

Delmi, M., Rapin, C.-H., Bengoa, J.M., Delmas, P.D., Vasey, H., Bonjour, J.P. (1990). Dietary supplementation in elderly patients with fractured neck of femur. *Lancet* **335**, 1013–1016.

Dempsey, D.T., Mullen, J.L. & Buzby, G.P. (1988). The link between nutritional status and clinical outcome. *Am. J. Clin. Nutr.* **47**, 352–356.

Demopoulos, H.B., Flamm, E.S., Pietronigro, D.D. & Seligman, M.L. (1980). The radical pathology and the microcirculation in the major central nervous system disorders. *Acta Physiol. Scand.* (Suppl) **492**, 91–119.

Demuth, K., Atger, V., Borderie, D., Benoit, M.O., Sauveget, D., Lotersztajn, S. & Moatti, N. (1999). Homocysteine decreases endothelin-1 production by cultured human endothelial cells. *Eur. J. Biochem.* **1263**, 367–376.

Department of Health and Social Security (1972). *Nutritional Survey of the Elderly*. Report on Public Health and Medical Subjects No. 3. HMSO, London.

Department of Health and Social Security (1979a). *Nutrition Survey of the Elderly*. Report on Health and Social Subjects No. 13. HMSO, London.

Department of Health and Social Security (1979b). *Nutrition and Health in Old Age*. Report on Health and Social Subjects No. 16. HMSO, London.

Department of Health and Social Security (1991). *Dietary Reference Values for Food Energy and Nutrients for the United Kingdom.* Report on Health and Social Subjects No. 41. HMSO London.

Department of Health and Social Security (1992). *Nutrition in the Elderly.* Report on Health and Social Subjects No. 43. HMSO, London.

Devaraj, S., Li, D. & Jialal, I.. (1996). The effects of alpha tocopherol supplementation on monocyte function. Decreased lipid oxidation, interleukin 1beta, and monocyte adhesion to endothelium. *J. Clin. Invest.* **98**, 756–763.

Dionigi, R., Dominioni, L., Jemos, V., Cremaschi, R. & Monico, R. (1986). Diagnosing malnutrition. *Gut* **27** (S1) 5–8.

Donahue, R.P., Abbott, R.D., Reed, D.M. & Yano, K. (1986). Alcohol and hemorrhagic stroke: The Honolulu Heart Program. *J. Am. Med. Assoc.* **255**, 2311–2314.

Drinka, P.J. & Goodwin, J.S. (1991). Prevalence and consequence of vitamin deficiency in nursing homes: a critical review. *J. Am. Geriatr. Soc.* **39**, 1008–1017.

Dudman, N.P., Temple, S.E., Guo, X.W., Fu, W. & Perry, M.A. (1999). Homocysteine enhances neutrophil–endothelial interactions in both cultured human cells and rats in vivo. *Circ. Res.* **84**, 409–416.

Durnin, J.V.G.A. (1961). Food intake and energy expenditure of elderly people. *Clin. Gerontol.* **4**, 128–133.

Durnin, J.V.G.A. (1985). Energy intake, energy expenditure and body composition in the elderly. In: *Nutrition, Immunity and Illness in the Elderly*, (Chandra, R.K., ed.), pp. 19–33. Pergamon Press, New York.

Durnin, J.V.G.A. & Lean, M.E.J. (1992). Nutrition – consideration for the elderly. In: *Textbook of Geriatric Medicine and Gerontology*, (Brocklehurst, J.C., Tallis, R.C. & Fillit, H.M., eds), pp. 592–610. Churchill Livingstone, London.

Durnin, J.V. & Womersley, S. (1974). Body fat assessed from total body density and its estimation from skinfold thickness: measurements on 481 men and women aged from 16 to 72 years. *Br. J. Nutr.* **32**, 77–97.

El Kossi, M.M.H. & Mahrous, Z.M. (2000). Oxidative stress in the context of acute cerebrovascular stroke. *Stroke* **31**, 1889–1892.

Elmstahl, S. & Steen, B. (1987). Hospital nutrition in geriatric long term care medicine: 11. Effects of dietary supplements. *Age Ageing* **16**, 73–80.

Enstrom, J.E., Kanim, L.E. & Klein, M.A. (1992). Vitamin C intake and mortality among a sample of the United States population. *Epidemiology* **3**, 194–202.

Euronut SENECA Investigators (1991). Nutritional status: blood vitamins A, E, B6, B12, folic acid and carotene. *Eur. J. Clin. Nutr.* **45**, 63–82.

Evans, E. & Stock, A.L. (1971). Dietary intake of geriatric patients in hospital. *Nutr. Metab.* **13**, 21–35.

Evans, R.W., Shaten, J., Hempel, J.D., Cutler, J.A. & Kuller, L.H. for the MRFIT Research Group (1997). Homocysteine and risk of cardiovascular disease in the Multiple Risk Factor Intervention Trial. *Arterioscler. Thromb. Vas. Biol.* **17**, 1947–1953.

Evans, S. & Fotherby, M.D. (1999). Cholesterol and stroke. *Rev. Clin. Gerontol.* **9**, 1–12.

Exton-Smith, A.N. (1980a). Nutritional status: diagnosis and prevention of malnutrition. In: *Metabolic and Nutritional Disorders in the Elderly*. (Exton-Smith, A.N. & Caird, F.I.. eds), pp. 66–76. John Wright & Sons, Bristol.

Exton-Smith, A.N. (1980b). Eating habits of the elderly. In: *Nutrition and Lifestyles*

(Proceedings of the British Nutrition Foundation, London, May 1979) (Turner, M. ed.) pp. 179–194. Applied Science Publishers, London.

Faruqi, R., de la Motte, C. & DiCorleto, P.E. (1994). Alpha-tocopherol inhibits agonist-induced monocytic cell adhesion to cultured human endothelial cells. *J. Clin. Invest.* **94**, 592–600.

Fassbender, K., Mossner, R., Motsch, L., Kischka, U., Grau, A. & Hennerici, M. (1995). Circulating selectin- and imunoglobulin-type adhesion molecules in acute ischaemic stroke. *Stroke* **26**, 1361–1364.

Feron, O., Dessy, C., Moniotte, S., Desager, J.P. & Balligand, J.L. (1999). Hypercholesterolemia decreases nitric oxide production by promoting the interaction of caveolin and endothelial nitric oxide synthase. *J. Clin. Invest.* **103**, 897–905.

Ferro-Luzzi, A., Mobarhan, S., Maiani, G., Scaccini, C., Sette, S. & Nicastro, A. (1988). Habitual alcohol consumption and nutritional status of the elderly. *Eur. J. Clin. Nutr.* **42**, 5–13.

Fiatarone, M.A., O'Neil, E.F., Ryan, N.D., Clements, K.M., Solares, G.R., Nelson, M.E., Roberts, S.B., Kehayias, J.J., Lipsitz, L.A. & Evans, W.J. (1994). Exercise training and nutritional supplementation for physical frailty in very elderly people. *New Engl. J. Med.* **330**, 1769–1775.

Finch, S., Doyle, W., Lowe, C., Bates, C., Prentice, A., Smithers, A. & Clarke, P. (1998). *National Diet and Nutrition Survey: People Aged 65 Years and Over. Volume I: Report of the Diet and Nutrition Survey.* Stationery Office, London.

Finkelstein, J.D. (1998). The metabolism of homocysteine: pathways and regulation. *Eur. J. Pediatr.* **157** (Suppl. 2), S40–S44.

Flamm, E.S., Demopoulos, H.B., Seligman, M.L., Posner, R.G. & Ransohoff, J. (1978). Radicals in cerebral ischaemia. *Stroke* **9**, 445–447.

Fleischhauer, F.J., Yan, W.D. & Fischell, T.A. (1993). Fish oil improves endothelium-dependent coronary vasodilation in heart transplant recipients. *J. Am. Coll. Cardiol.* **21**, 982–989.

Fletcher, G.F. (1994). Exercise in the prevention of stroke. *Health Rep.* **6**, 106–110.

Folsom, A.R., Nieto, J., McGovern, P.G., Tsai, M.Y., Malinow, M.R., Eckfeldt, J.H., Hess, D.L. & Davis, C.E. (1998). Prospective study of coronary heart disease incidence in relation to fasting total homocysteine, related genetic pleomorphism and B vitamins (ARIC Study). *Circulation* **98**, 204–210.

Folsom, A.R., Rasmussen, M.L., Chambless, L.E., Howard, G., Cooper, L.S., Schmidt, M.I. & Heiss, G. (1999). Prospective associations of fasting insulin, body fat distribution, and diabetes with risk of ischaemic stroke. *Diabetes Care* **22**(7), 1077–1083.

Fontana, L., McNeill, K.L., Ritter, J.M. & Chowienczyk, P.J. (1999). Effects of vitamin C and of a cell permeable superoxide dismutase mimetic on acute lipoprotein induced endothelial dysfunction in rabbit aortic rings. *Br. J. Pharmacol.* **120**, 730–734.

FOOD Trial Collaboration (2003). Poor nutritional status on admission predicts poor outcome after stroke: observational data from the FOOD trial. *Stroke* **34**(6), 1450–1456.

Forbes, G.B. & Reina, J.C. (1970). Adult lean body mass declines with age: some longitudinal observations. *Metabolism* **19**, 653–663.

Forbes, J.F. (1993). Cost of stroke. *Scottish Med. J.* **38**(3 Suppl.), S4–S5.

Fotherby, M.D. & Potter, J.F. (1993). Potassium supplementation reduces clinic and ambulatory blood pressure in elderly hypertensive patients. *J. Hypertension* **10**(11), 1403–1408.

Frankel, E.N., Parks, E.J., Xu, R., Schneeman, B.O., Davis, P.A. & German, J.B. (1994). Effect of n-3 fatty acid-rich fish oil supplementation on the oxidation of low density lipoproteins. *Lipids* **29**, 233–236.

Frantzen, F., Faaren, A.L., Alfheim, I. & Nordhei, A.K. (1998). Enzyme conversion immunoassay for determining total homocysteine in plasma or serum. *Clin. Chem.* **44**, 311–316.

Freeman, B.A., Young, S.L. & Crapo, J.D. (1983). Liposome-mediated augmentation of superoxide dismutase in endothelial cells prevents oxygen injury. *J. Biol. Chem.* **258**, 12534–12542.

Fridovich, I. (1986). Biological effects of the superoxide radical. *Arch. Biochem. Biophys.* **247**, 1–11.

Friedenreich, C.M., Slimani, N. & Riboli, E. (1992). Measurement of past diet: review of previous and proposed methods. *Epidemiol. Rev.* **14**, 177–195.

Friedmann, J.M., Jensen, G.L., Smiciklas-Wright, H. & McCamish, M.A. (1997). Predicting early nonelective hospital readmission in nutritionally compromised older adults. *Am. J. Clin. Nutr.* **65**, 1714–1720.

Frijns, C.J.M., Kappelle, L.J., van Gign, J., Nieuwenhuis, H.K., Sixma, J.J. & Fijnheer, R. (1997). Soluble adhesion molecules reflect endothelial cell activation in ischaemic stroke and in carotid atherosclerosis. *Stroke* **28**, 2214–2218.

Frisancho, A.R. (1984). New standard of body weight and composition by frame size and height for assessment of nutritional status of adults and elderly. *Am. J. Clin. Nutr.* **40**, 808–819.

Frosman, M., Fleischer, J.E., Milde, J.H., Steen, P.A. & Michenfelder, J.D. (1988). Superoxide dismutase and catalase failed to improve neurological outcome after complete cerebral ischaemia in the dog. *Acta Anaesthesiol. Scand.* **32**, 152–155.

Frosst, P., Blom, H.J., Milos, R., Goyette, P., Sheppard, C.A., Matthews, R.G., Boers, G.J., den Heijer, M., Kluytmans, L.A. & van den Heuvel, L.P. (1995). Candidate genetic risk factor for vascular disease: a common mutation in methyltetrahydrofolate reductase. *Nat. Genet.* **10**, 111–113.

Fuller, N.J., Sawyer, M.B., Laskey, M.A., Paxton, P. & Elia, M. (1996). Prediction of body composition in elderly men over 75 years of age. *Ann. Hum. Biol.* **23**(2), 127–147.

Gale, C.R., Martyn, C.N., Winter, P.D. & Cooper, C. (1995). Vitamin C and risk of death from stroke and coronary heart disease in cohort of elderly people. *Br. Med. J.* **310**, 1563–1566.

Gariballa, S.E. (1998). *Nutritional status and outcomes after acute stroke*. Doctoral thesis (MD), Leicester, G2h, 48–9117.

Gariballa, S.E. (2000). Nutritional factors in stroke. *Br. J. Nutr.* **84**, 5–17.

Gariballa, S.E. (2001). Malnutrition in hospitalised elderly patients: when does it matter? *Clin. Nutr.* **20**(6), 487–491.

Gariballa, S.E. (2002). Potentially treatable causes of poor outcome in acute stroke patients with urinary incontinence. *Acta Neurol. Scand.* **107**(5), 336–340.

Gariballa, S.E. & Sinclair, A.J. (1998a). Nutrition, ageing and ill health. *Br. J. Nutr.* **80**(1), 7–23.

Gariballa, S.E. & Sinclair, A.J. (1998b). Assessment and treatment of nutritional status in stroke patients. *Postgrad. Med. J.* **74**, 395–399.

Gariballa, S.E. & Sinclair, A.J. (1999). Oxidative stress and cerebrovascular disease. *Rev. Clin. Gerontol.* **9**, 197–206.

Gariballa, S.E., Robinson, T.G. & Fotherby, M.D. (1997). Hypokalaemia and potassium excretion in stroke patients. *J. Am. Geriatr. Soc.* **45**, 1454–1458.

Gariballa, S.E., Taub, N., Parker, S.G. & Castleden, C.M. (1998a). A randomised controlled trial of oral nutritional supplements following acute stroke. *J. Parent. Ent. Nutr.* **22**, 315–319.

Gariballa, S.E., Taub, N., Parker, S.G. & Castleden, C.M. (1998b). Nutritional status of hospitalised acute stroke patients. *Br. J. Nutr.* **79**, 481–487.

Gariballa, S.E., Taub, N., Parker, S.G. & Castleden, C.M. (1998c). The influence of nutritional status on clinical outcome after acute stroke. *Am. J. Clin. Nutr.* **68**, 275–281.

Gariballa, S.G., Hutchin, T. & Sinclair, A.J. (2002). Antioxidant capacity after acute stroke. *Q. J. Med.* **95**, 685–690.

Garrow, J. (1994). Starvation in hospital. *Br. Med. J.* **308**, 934 (abstract).

Garrow, J.S., James, W.P.T. & Ralph, A. (2000). *Human Nutrition and Dietetics.* 10th edn, Ch. 42. Churchill Livingstone, Edinburgh.

Garth, S. & Young, R. (1956). Concurrent fat loss and fat gain. *Am. J. Phys. Anthropol.* **14**, 497–504.

Gaudet, R.J., Alam, I. & Levine, L. (1980). Accumulation of cycloxygenase products of arachidonic acid metabolism in gerbil brain during reperfusion after bilateral common carotid artery occlusion. *J. Neurochem.* **35**, 653–658.

Geissler, C.A. & Bates, J.F. (1984). The nutritional effects of tooth loss. *Am. J. Clin. Nutr.* **39**, 478–489.

Gey, K.F., Moser, U.K., Jordan, P., Stahelin, H.B., Eichholzer, M. & Ludin, E. (1993a). Increased risk of cardiovascular disease at suboptimal plasma conentration of essential antioxidants. *Am. J. Clin. Nutr.* **57**(Suppl.), 787S–797S.

Gey, K.F., Stahelin, H.B. & Eichholzer, M. (1993b). Poor plasma status of carotene and vitamin C is associated with higher mortality from ischaemic heart disease and stroke. *Clin. Invest.* **71**, 3–6.

Giles, W.H., Kittner, S.J., Anda, R.F., Croft, J.B. & Casper, M.L. (1995). Serum folate and risk for ischaemic stroke. *Stroke* **26**, 1166–1170.

Giles, W.H., Croft, J.B., Greenlund, K.J., Ford, E.S. & Kittner, S.J. (1998). Total homocysteine concentration and the likelihood of nonfatal stroke: results from the Third National Health and Nutritional Survey, 1988–1994. *Stroke* **29**, 2473–2477.

Gill, J.S., Zezulka, A.V., Shipley, M.J., Gill, S.K. & Beevers, D.G. (1986). Stroke and alcohol consumption. *N. Engl. J. Med.* **315**, 1041–1046.

Gillman, M.W., Cupples, L.A., Gagnon, D., Posner, B.M., Ellison, R.C., Castelli, W.P. & Wolf, P.A. (1995). Protective effect of fruits and vegetables on development of stroke in men. *J. Am. Med. Assoc.* **273**(14), 1113–1117.

Gillman, M.W., Cupples, L.A., Millen, B.E., Ellison, R.C. & Wolfe, P.A. (1997). Inverse association of dietary fat with development of ischaemic stroke in men. *J. Am. Med. Assoc.* **278**, 2145–2150.

Gillum, R.F. & Makuc, D.M. (1992). Serum albumin, coronary heart disease and death. *Am. Heart J.* **123**, 507–513.

Gillum, R.F., Ingram, D.D. & Makuc, D.M. (1994). Relation between serum albumin concentration and stroke incidence and death: The NHANES 1 Epidemiologic Follow-up Study. *Am. J. Epidemiol.* **140**, 876–888.

Gillum, R.F., Mussolino, M.E. & Madans, J.H. (1996). The NHANES 1 Epidemiologic Follow-up Study. *Arch. Inter. Med.* **156**, 537–542.

GISSI-Prevenzione Investigators (1999). Dietary supplementation with n-3 poly-unsaturated fatty acids and vitamin E after myocardial infarction: results from the GISSI-Prevenzione trial. *Lancet* **354**, 447–455.

Gocke, N., Keaney, J.F., Frei, B., Holbrook, M., Olesiak, M., Zachariah, B.J., Leeu-wenburgh, C., Heinecke, J.W. & Vita, J.A. (1999). Long-term ascorbic acid adminis-tration reverses endothelial vasomotor dysfunction in patients with coronary artery disease. *Circulation* **99**, 3234–3240.

Golden, M.H.N. & Waterlow, J.C. (1977). Total protein synthesis in elderly people: a comparison of results with ^{15}N glycine and ^{14}C leucine. *Clin. Sci. Mol. Med.* **53**, 277–288.

Goldman, L. & Cook, E.F. (1984). The decline in ischaemic heart disease mortality rates. An analysis of the comparative effects of medical intervention and changes in life-style. *Ann. Intern. Med.* **101**, 825–836.

Goodfellow, J., Bellamy, M.F., Ramsey, M.W., Jones, C.J. & Lewis, M.J. (2000). Dietary supplementation with marine omega-3 fatty acids improves systemic large artery endothelial function in subjects with hypercholesterolemia. *J. Am. Coll. Cardiol.* **35**, 265–270.

Gordon, C., Langton Hewer, R. & Wade, D.T. (1987). Dysphagia in acute stroke. *Br. Med. J.* **295**, 411–414.

Gordon, T., Garcia-Palmieri, M.R., Kagan, A., Kannel, W.B. & Schiffman, J. (1974). Differences in coronary heart disease in Honolulu and Puerto Rico. *J. Chron. Dis.* **27**, 329–344.

Gorelick, P.B. (1989). The status of alcohol as a risk factor for stroke. *Stroke* **20**, 1607–1610.

Gorelick, P.B., Sacco, R.L., Smith, D.B., Alberts, M., Mustone-Alexander, L., Rader, D. Ross, D.L., Raps, E., Ozer, M.N., Brass, L.M. et al. (1999). Prevention of a first stroke: a review of guidelines and multidisciplinary consensus statement from the National Stroke Association. *J. Am. Med. Assoc.* **281**(12), 1112–1120.

Graham, I.M., Daly, L.E., Refsum, H.M., Robinson, K., Brattstrom, L.E., Ueland, P.M., Palma Reis, R.J., Boers, G.H., Sheaham, R.G., Israelsson, B. et al. (1997). Plasma homocysteine as a risk factor for vascular disease. The European Concerted Action Project. *J. Am. Med. Assoc.* **277**, 1775–1781.

Gregory, J., Foster, K., Tyler, H. & Wiseman, M. (1990). *The Dietary and Nutritional Survey of British Adults.* HMSO, London.

Guigoz, Y., Vellas, B. & Garry, P.J. (1994). Mini nutritional assessment. In: *Nutrition in the Elderly* (Vellas, B.J., Guigoz, Y., Garry, P.J., Albarede, J.L., eds), Supplement 2, pp. 15–32. Serdi, Paris.

Gupta, K.L., Dworkin, B. & Gambert, S.R. (1988). Common nutritional disorders in the elderly: atypical manifestations. *Geriatrics* **43**(2), 87–97.

Guttormsen, A.B., Scheede, J., Fiskerstrand, T., Ueland, P.M. & Refsum, H.M. (1994). Plasma concentrations of homocysteine and other aminothiol compounds are related to food intake in healthy human subjects. *J. Nutr.* **124**, 1934–1941.

Haboubi, N.Y. & Montgomery, R.D. (1992). Small bowel bacterial overgrowth in elderly people: clinical significance and response to treatment. *Age Ageing* **21**, 13–19.

Haley, E.C. (1998). High dose tirilazad for acute stroke (RANTTAS II). *Stroke* **29**, 1256–1257.

Hallenbeck, J.M. & Furlow, T.W. (1979). Prostaglandins I_2 and indomethacin prevent impairment of post-ischaemic brain reperfusion in the dog. *Stroke* **10**, 629–637.

Hallenbeck, J.M., Dutka, A.J., Tanishima, T., Kochanek, P.M., Kumaroo, K.K., Thompson, C.B., Obrenovitch, T.P. & Contreras, T.J. (1986). Polymorphonuclear leukocyte accumulation in brain regions with low blood flow during the early postischaemic period. *Stroke* **17**, 246–253.

Halliwell, B. (1989). Oxidants and the central nervous system: some fundamental questions. *Acta Neurol. Scand.* **126**, 23–33.

Halliwell, B. (1994). Free radicals, antioxidants, and human disease: curiosity, cause or consequence? *Lancet* **344**, 721–724.

Halliwell, B. (2000). The antioxidants paradox. *Lancet* **355**, 1179–1180.

Halliwell, B. & Gutteridge, J.M.C. (1984) Oxygen toxicity, oxygen radicals, transition metals and disease. *Biochemistry* **219**, 1–14.

Halliwell, B. & Gutteridge, J. (1985). Oxygen radicals and the nervous system. *Trends Neurosci.* **8**, 22–26.

Hambrecht, R., Wolf, A., Gielen, S., Linke, A., Hofer, J., Erbs, S., Schone, N. & Schuler, G. (2000). Effect of exercise on coronary endothelial function in patients with coronary artery disease. *N. Engl. J. Med.* **342**, 454–460.

Hankey, G.J. & Eikelboom, J.W. (1999). Homocysteine and vascular disease. *Lancet* **354**, 407–413.

Hankey, C.R., Summerbell, J. & Wynne, H.A. (1993). The effect of dietary supplementation in continuing care of elderly people. *J. Hum. Nutr. Diet.* **6**, 317–322.

Harker, L.A., Ross, R., Slichter, S.J. & Scott, C.R. (1976). Homocystine-induced arteriosclerosis: the role of endothelial cell injury and platelet response in its genesis. *J. Clin. Invest.* **58**, 731–741.

Harker, L.A., Harlan, J.M. & Ross, R. (1983). Effect of sulfinpyrazone on homocysteine-induced endothelial injury and arteriosclerosis in baboons. *Circ. Res.* **53**, 731–739.

Harris, W.S. (1989). Fish oils and plasma lipid and lipoprotein metabolism in humans: a critical review. *J. Lipid Res.* **30**, 785–807.

Hartz, S.C., Roenberg, I.H. & Russel, R.M. (1992). *Nutrition in the Elderly. The Boston Nutritional Survey*. Smith Gordon, London.

Haynes, W.G. (1999). Vascular effects of homocysteine: therapeutic implications. *Heart Failure* **15**, 153–163.

Heaney, R.P., Gallagher, J.C., Johnston, C.C., Neer, R., Parfitt, A.M. & Whedon, G.D. (1982). Calcium nutrition and bone health in the elderly. *Am. J. Clin. Nutr.* **36**, 986–1013.

Heart Protection Study Collaborative Group (2002). MRC/BHF heart protection study of antioxidant vitamin supplementation in 20 536 high-risk individuals: a randomised placebo-controlled trial. *Lancet* **360**, 23–33.

Heber, D. & Bray, G.A. (1980). Energy requirements. In: *Metabolic and Nutritional Dis-*

orders in the Elderly (Exton-Smith, A.N. & Caird, F.I. eds), pp. 1–12. John Wright & Sons, Bristol.

Hebert, P.R., Gaziano, J.M. & Hennekens, C.H. (1995). An overview of trials of cholesterol lowering and risk of stroke. *Arch. Int. Med.* **155**, 50–55.

Heinecke, J.W., Kawamura, M., Suzuki, L. & Chait, A. (1993). Oxidation of low density lipoprotein by thiols: superoxide-dependent and -independent mechanisms. *J. Lipid Res.* **34**, 2051–2061.

Heiss, W.-D. & Graf, R. (1994). The ischaemic penumbra. *Curr. Opin. Neurol.* **7**, 11–19.

Heitzer, T., Just, H. & Munzel, T. (1996). Antioxidant vitamin C improves endothelial dysfunction in chronic smokers. *Circulation* **94**, 6–9.

Hennekens, C.H., Buring, J.E., Manson, J.E., Stamper, M., Posner, B., Cook, N.R., Belanger, C., LaMotte, F., Gaziano, J.M., Ridker, P.M. et al. (1996). Lack of effect of long-term supplementation with beta carotene on the incidence of malignant neoplasm and cardiovascular disease. *New Engl. J. Med.* **334**, 1145–1149.

Herbert, P.R., Gaziano, J.M., Chan, K.S. & Hennekens, C.H. (1997). Cholesterol lowering with statin drugs, risk of stroke, and total mortality. *J. Am. Med. Assoc.* **278**, 313–321.

Heyland, D.K., MacDonald, S., Keefe, L. & Drover, J.W. (1998). Total parenteral nutrition in critically ill patients. *J. Am. Med. Assoc.* **280**, 2013–2019.

Higman, D.J., Strachan, A.M., Buttery, L., Hicks, R.C., Springall, D.R., Greenhalgh, R.M. & Powell, J.T. (1996). Smoking impairs the activity of endothelial nitric oxide synthase in saphenous vein. *Arterioscler. Thromb. Vasc. Biol.* **16**, 546–552.

Hoffman, N. (1993). Diet in the elderly: needs and risk. *Clin. Nutr.* **77**, 745–756.

Holven, K.B., Holm, T., Aukrust, P., Christensen, B., Kjekshus, J., Andreassen, A.K., Gullestad, L., Hagve, T.A., Svilaas, A., Ose, L. & Nenseter, M.S. (2001). Effect of folic acid treatment on endothelium-dependent vasodilation and nitric oxide-derived end products in hyperhomocysteinaemic subjects. *Am. J. Med.* **110**(7), 536–542.

Homocysteine Lowering Trialists' Collaboration (1998). Lowering blood homocysteine with folic acid based supplements: meta-analysis of randomised trials. *Br. Med. J.* **316**, 894–898.

Hornig, B., Arakawa, N., Kohler, C. & Drexler, H. (1998). Vitamin C improves endothelial function of conduit arteries in patients with chronic heart failure. *Circulation* **97**, 363–368.

Horwath, C.C. (1993). Validity of a short food frequency questionnaire for estimating nutrient intake in elderly people. *Br. J. Nutr.* **70**, 3–14.

Houston, P.E., Rana, S., Sekhsaria, S., Perlin, E., Kim, K.S. & Castro, O.L. (1997). Homocysteine in sickle cell disease: relationship to stroke. *Am. J. Med.* **103**(3), 192–196.

Howard, L., Dillon, B., Saba, T.M., Hofmann, S. & Cho, E. (1984). Decreased plasma fibronectin during starvation in man. *J. Parent. Ent. Nutr.* **8**, 237–244.

Howard, V.H., Sides, E.G., Newman, G.C., Cohen, S.N., Howard, G., Malinow, M.R. & Toole, J.F. (2000). Changes in plasma homocysteine in the acute phase after stroke. *Stroke* **33**, 473–478.

Hu, F.B. & Stampfer, M.J. (1999). Nut consumption and risk of coronary heart disease: a review of epidemiologic evidence. *Curr. Atherosclerosis Rep.* **1**, 204–209.

Hu, F.B., Stampfer, M.J., Manson, J.E., Rimm, E., Colditz, G.A., Speizer, F.E., Hennekens, C.H. & Willet, W.C. (1999a). Dietary protein and risk of ischemic heart disease in women. *Am. J. Clin. Nutr.* **70**, 221–227.

Hu, F.B., Stampfer, M.J., Colditz, G.A., Ascherio, A., Rexrode, K.M., Willett, W.C. & Manson, J.E. (2000). Physical activity and risk of stroke in women. *J. Am. Med. Assoc.* **283**(22), 2961–2967.

Hu, F.B., Stampfer, M.J., Solomon, C., Liu, S., Colditz, G.A., Speizer, F.E., Willett, W.C. & Manson, J.E. (2001). Physical activity and risk for cardiovascular events in diabetic women. *Ann. Int. Med.* **134**(2), 96–105.

Hwang, S., Ballantyne, C., Sharrett, R., Smith, L.C., Davis, C.E., Gotto, A.M. Jr & Boerwinkle, E. (1997). Circulating adhesion molecules VCAM-1, ICAM-1, and E-selectin in carotid atherosclerosis and incident coronary heart disease cases: the Atherosclerosis Risk in Communities (ARIC) Study. *Circulation* **96**, 4219–4225.

Iansek, R., Packham, D., Aspey, B.S. & Harrison, M.J.G. (1986). An assessment of the possible protective effect of allopurinol in acute stroke. *FEBS Lett.* **213**, 23–28.

Imaizumi, S.T., Kayama, T. & Suzuki, J. (1984). Chemiluminescence in hypoxic brain – the first report. *Stroke* **15**, 1061–1065.

Imaizumi, S., Woolworth, V., Fishman, R.A. & Chan, P.H. (1990). Liposome entrapped superoxide dismutase reduces cerebral infarction in cerebral ischemia in rats. *Stroke* **21**, 1312–1317.

Intersalt Cooperative Research Group (1988) An international study of electrolyte excretion and blood pressure. Results for 24 hour urinary sodium and potassium excretion. *Br. Med. J.* **297**, 319–328.

Iso, H., Rexrode, K.M., Stampfer, M.J., Manson, J.E., Colditz, G.A., Speizer, F.E., Hennekens, C.H. & Willett, W.C. (2001). Intake of fish and omega-3 fatty acids and risk of stroke in women. *J. Am. Med. Assoc.* **285**(3), 304–312.

Jacques, P.F., Selhub, J., Bostom, A.G., Wilson, P.W. & Rosenberg, I.H. (1999). The effect of folic acid fortification on plasma folate and total homocysteine concentrations. *New Engl. J. Med.* **340**, 1449–1454.

Johansen, O., Seljflot, I., Hostmark, A.T. & Arnesen, H. (1999). The effect of supplementation with omega-3 fatty acids on soluble markers of endothelial function in patients with coronary heart disease. *Arterioscler. Thromb. Vasc. Biol.* **19**, 1681–1686.

Jones, T.H., Morawetz, R.B. & Crowell, R.M. (1981). Threshold of focal cerebral ischaemia in awake monkeys. *J. Neurosurg.* **54**, 773–782.

Joosten, E., Berg, A.V.D., Reizler, R., Naurath, H.J. & Lindenbaum, J. (1993). Metabolic evidence that deficiencies of vitamin B12, folate and vitamin B6 occur commonly in elderly people. *Am. J. Clin. Nutr.* **58**, 468–476.

Kagan, A., Popper, J.S., Rhoads, G.G. & Yano, K. (1985). Dietary and other risk factors for stroke in Hawaiian Japanese men. *Stroke* **16**(3), 390–396.

Kang, J.X. & Leaf, A. (2000). Prevention of fatal cardiac arrhythmias by polyunsaturated fatty acids. *Am. J. Clin. Nutr.* **71**(Suppl), 202S–207S.

Kang, S.S., Wong, P.W.K. & Norusis, M. (1987). Homocysteinaemia due to folate deficiency. *Metabolism* **36**, 458–462.

Kang, S.S., Zhou, J., Wong, P.W.R., Kowalisyn, J. & Strokosch, G. (1988). Intermediate homocysteinaemia: a thermolabile variant of methyltetrahydrofolate reductase. *Am. J. Hum. Genet.* **43**, 414–421.

Keli, S.O., Hertog, M.G.L., Feskens, E.J.M. & Kromhout, D. (1996). Dietary flavonoids, antioxidant vitamins, and incidence of stroke. *Arch. Int. Med.* **154**, 637–642.

Keller, H.H. (1995). Weight gain impacts morbidity and mortality in institutionalised older persons. *J. Am. Geriatr. Soc.* **43**, 165–169.

Kempski, O., Shohami, E., von Lubitz, D., Hallenbeck, J.M. & Feuerstein, G. (1987). Postischaemic production of eicosanoids in gerbil brain. *Stroke* **18**, 111–119.

Khalfoun, B., Thibault, G., Bardos, P. & Lebranchu, Y. (1996). Docosahexaenoic and eicosapentaenoic acids inhibit in vitro human lymphocyte–endothelial adhesion. *Transplantation* **62**, 1649–1657.

Khaw, K.T. & Barrett-Connor, E. (1987). Dietary potassium and stroke associated mortality. A 12-year prospective population study. *New Engl. J. Med.* **316**(5), 235–239.

Kim, P., Yaksh, T.L., Burnett, P.C., Blum, M.R. & Sundt, T.M. (1987). Cerebrovascular fluid levels of uric acid in dogs and the effect of allopurinol. *Brain Res.* **402**, 87–92.

Kimoto-Kinoshita, S., Nishida, S. & Tomura, T.T. (1999). Age-related change of antioxidant capacities in the cerebral cortex and hippocampus of stroke-prone spontaneously hypertensive rats. *Neurosci. Lett.* **273**(1), 41–44.

Kimura, N., Toshima, H., Nakayama, Y., Mizuguchi, T. & Fukami, T. (1972). Population survey on cerebrovascular and cardiovascular diseases. The ten years experience in the farming village of Tanuschimaru and the fishing village of Ushibuka. *Jpn. Heart J.* **13**(2), 118–127.

Kipstein-Grobusch, K., Reilly, J.J., Potter, J., Edwards, C.A. & Roberts, M.A. (1995). Energy intake and expenditure in elderly patients admitted to hospital with acute illness. *Br. J. Nutr.* **73**, 323–334.

Klein, S., Kinney, J., Jeejeebhoy, K., Alpers, D., Hellerstein, M., Murray, M. & Twomey, P. (1997). Nutrition support in clinical practice: review of published data. *Am. J. Clin. Nutr.* **66**, 683–706.

Klidjian, A.M., Archer, T.J. & Foster, K.J. (1982). Detection of dangerous malnutrition. *J. Parent. Ent. Nutr.* **6**, 119–123.

Knekt, P., Reunanen, A., Jarvinen, R., Seppanen, R., Heliovaara, M. & Aromma, A. (1994). Antioxidant vitamin intake and coronary mortality in a longitudinal population study. *Am. J. Epidemiol.* **139**, 1180–1189.

Knight, I. & Eldridge, J. (1984). *The Heights and Weights of Adults in Great Britain*. HMSO, London.

Kocaturk, P.A., Akbostanci, M.C., Isikay, C., Ocal, A., Tuncel, D., Kavas, G.O. & Mutluer, N. (2001). Antioxidant status in cerebrovascular accident. *Biol. Trace Elem. Res.* **80**(2), 115–124.

Kochanek, P.M., Dutka, A.J. & Hallenbeck, J.M. (1987). Indomethacin, prostacyclin and heparin improve postischaemic cerebral blood flow without affecting early postischaemic granulocyte accumulation. *Stroke* **18**, 634–637.

Kokkinos, P.F., Narayan, P., Colleran, J.A., Pittaras, A., Notargiacomo, A., Reda, A. & Papademetriou, V. (1995). Effects of regular exercise on blood pressure and left ventricular hypertrophy in African-American men with severe hypertension. *New Engl. J. Med.* **333**, 1462–1467.

Kontos, H.A., Wei, E.P., Ellis, E.F., Jenkins, L.W., Povlishock, J.T., Rowe, G.T. & Hess, M.L. (1985). Appearance of superoxide anion radical in cerebral extracellular space during increased prostaglandin synthesis in cats. *Circ. Res.* **57**, 142–151.

Kotler, D.P., Wang, J. & Pierson, R.N. Jr. (1985). Body composition studies in patients with the acquired immunodeficiency syndrome. *Am. J. Clin. Nutr.* **42**, 1255–1265.

Kugiyama, K., Motoyama, T., Doi, H., Kawano, H., Hirani, N., Soejima, H., Miyao, Y., Takazoe, K., Moriyama, Y., Mizuno, Y. et al. (1999). Improvement of endothelial vasomotor dysfunction by treatment with alpha-tocopherol in patients with high remnant lipoprotein levels. *J. Am. Coll. Cardiol.* **33**, 1512–1518.

Kuhn, F.E., Mohler, E.R., Salter, L.F., Reagan, K., Lu, D.Y. & Rackley, C.E. (1991). Effects of high density lipoprotein on acetylcholine-induced coronary vasoreactivity. *Am. J. Cardiol.* **68**, 1425–1430.

Kuller, L.H., Eichner, J.E, Orchard, T.J., Grandits, G.A., McCullum, L. & Tracy, R.P. (1991). The relation between serum albumin levels and risk of coronary heart disease in the multiple risk factor intervention trial. *Am. J. Epidemiol.* **134**, 1266–1277.

Kushi, L.H., Folsom, A.R., Prineas, R.J., Mink, P.J., Wu, Y. & Bostick, R.M. (1996). Dietary antioxidant vitamins and death from coronary heart disease in post-menopausal women. *New Engl. J. Med.* **334**, 115–162.

Kwok, T. & Whitelaw, M.N. (1991). The use of armspan in nutritional assessment of the elderly. *J. Am. Geriatr. Soc.* **39**, 492–496.

Lake, C.R., Ziegler, M.G., Coleman, M.D. & Kopin, I.J. (1977). Age-adjusted plasma norepinephrine levels are similar in normotensive and hypertensive subjects. *New Engl. J. Med.* **296**, 208–209.

Lakka, T.A. & Salonen, J.T. (1993). Moderate to high intensity conditioning leisure time physical activity and high cardiorespiratory fitness are associated with reduced plasma fibrinogen in eastern Finnish men. *J. Clin. Epidemiol.* **46**, 1119–1127.

Lampl, Y., Fleminger, G., Gilad, R., Galron, R., Sarova-Pinhas, I. & Sokolovsky, M. (1997). Endothelin in cerebrospinal fluid and plasma of patients in the early stage of ischaemic stroke. *Stroke* **28**(10), 1951–1955.

Langford, H.G. (1983). Dietary potassium and hypertension: epidemiologic data. *Ann. Int. Med.* **98**, 770–772.

Larsson, J., Unosson, M., Ek, A.C., Nilsson, L., Thorslund S. & Bjurulf, P. (1990). Effect of dietary supplement on nutritional status and clinical outcome in 501 geriatric patients. *Clin. Nutr.* **9**, 179–184.

Lehmann, A.B., Johnston, C. & James, O.F.W. (1989). The effects of old age and immobility on protein turnover in human subjects with some observations on possible role of hormones. *Age Ageing* **18**, 148–157.

Leinonen, J.S., Ahonen, J.P., Lonnrot, K., Jehkonen, M., Dastidar, P.P., Molnar, G. & Alho H.L. (2000). Plasma antioxidant activity is associated with high lesion volume and neurological impairment in stroke. *Stroke* **31**, 33–39.

Lennard-Jones, J.E. (1992). *A Positive Approach to Nutrition as Treatment*. King's Fund, London.

Lennard-Jones, J.E. (1999). Giving or withholding fluids and nutrients: ethical and legal aspects. *J. R. Coll. of Physicians London* **33**, 39-45.

Lentz, S.R., Sobey, C.G., Piegors, D.J., Bhopatkar, M.Y., Faraci, F.M., Malinow, M.R. & Heistad, D.D. (1996). Vascular dysfunction in monkeys with diet-induced hyperhomocyst(e)inemia. *J. Clin. Invest.* **98**, 24–29.

Lerman, A., Burnett, J.C., Higano, S.T., McKinley, L.J. & Holmes, D.R. (1998). Long-term L-arginine supplementation improves small vessel coronary endothelial function in humans. *Circulation* **97**, 2123–2128.

Lim, K.H., Connolly, M., Rose, D., Sridhar, F., Jacobowitz, I., Acinapura, A. & Cunningham, J.M. (1986). Prevention of reperfusion injury of the ischaemic spinal cord: use of recombinant superoxide dismutase. *Ann. Thor. Surg.* **42**, 282–286.

Lindenstrom, E., Boysen, G. & Nyboe, J. (1994). Influence of total cholesterol, HDL and triglyceride on risk of cerebrovascular disease. *Br. Med. J.* **309**,11–15.

Lindgren, A., Brattstrom, L., Novrrving, B., Hultberg, B., Andersson, A. & Johansson, B.B. (1995). Plasma homocysteine in the acute and convalescent phases after stroke. *Stroke* **26**(5), 795–800.

Lindsberg, P.J., Carpen, O., Paetau, A., Karjalainen-Lindsberg, M.L. & Kaste, M. (1996). Endothelial ICAM-1 expression associated with inflammatory cell response in human ischaemic stroke. *Circulation* **94**, 939–945.

Lip, G.Y.H., Blann, A.D., Farooqi, I.S., Zarifis, J., Sagar, G. & Beevers, D.G. (2001). Abnormal haemorrheology, endothelial function and thrombogenesis in relation to hypertension in acute (ictus <12h) stroke patients: The West Birmingham Stroke Project. *Blood Coag. Fibrin* **12**(4), 307–315.

Lipski, P.S., Kelly, P.J. & James, O.F.W. (1992). Bacterial contamination of the small bowel in elderly people: is it necessarily pathological? *Age Ageing* **21**, 5–12.

Liu, S., Manson, J.E., Stampfer, M.J., Rexrode, K.M., Hu, F.B., Rimm, E.B. & Willett, W.C. (2000). Whole grain consumption and risk of ischemic stroke in women: a prospective study. *J. Am. Med. Assoc.* **284**(12), 1534–1540.

Lo, W.D. & Betz, A.L. (1986). Oxygen free radical reduction of brain capillary rubidium uptake. *J. Neurochem.* **46**, 394–398.

Loenen, H.M.J.A., Eshuis, H., Lowik, M.R.H., Schouten, E.G., Hulshof, K.F., Odink, J. & Kok, F.J. (1990). Serum uric acid correlates in elderly men and women with special reference to body composition and dietary intake. *J. Clin. Epidemiol.* **43**, 1297–1303.

Lonergan, M.E. Milne, J.S., Malue, M.M. & Williamson, J. (1975). A dietary survey of older people in Edinburgh. *Br. J. Nutr.* **34**, 517–526.

Lonn, E.M. & Yusuf, S. (1999). Emerging approaches in preventing cardiovascular disease. *Br. Med. J.*, **318**, 1337–1341.

Losonczy, K.G., Harris, T.B. & Havlik, R.J. (1996). Vitamin E and vitamin C supplement use and risk of all-cause and coronary heart disease mortality in older persons: the Established Populations for Epidemiologic Studies of the Elderly. *Am. J. Clin. Nutr.* **64**,190–196.

Lundgren, B.K., Steen, B. & Isaksson, B. (1987). Dietary habits in 70- and 75-year old males and females. Longitudinal and cohort data from a population study. *Naringforskning* **31**, 53–56.

McCully, K.S. (1969). Vascular pathology of homocysteinaemia: implications for the pathogensis of atherosclerosis. *Am. J. Pathol.* **56**, 111–128.

McCully, K.S. (1996). Homocysteine and vascular disease. *Nat. Med.* **12**, 386–389.

McDowell, I.F. & Lang, D. (2000). Homocysteine and endothelial dysfunction: a link with cardiovascular disease. *J. Nutr.* **130**, 369S–372S.

McEvoy, A., Dutton, J. & James, O.F.W. (1983). Bacterial contamination of the small intestine is an important cause of occult malabsorption in the elderly. *Br. Med. J.* **287**, 789–793.

McGandy, R.B., Barrows, C.H., Spanias, C.H., Meredith, A., Stone, J.L. & Norris, A.H. (1966). Nutrient intake and energy expenditure in men of different ages. *J. Gerontol.* **21**, 581–587.

McGee, D., Reed, D., Stemmerman, G., Rhoads, G., Yano, K. & Feinleib, M. (1985). The relationship of dietary fat and cholesterol to mortality in 10 years. *Int. J. Epidemiol.* **14**(1), 97–105.

MacGregor, G.A. (1983). Sodium and potassium intake and the blood pressure. *Hypertension* **5**, 79–84.

McNamara, E.P., Flood, & P. Kennedy, N.P. (2000). Enteral tube feeding in the community: survey of adult patients discharged from a Dublin hospital. *Clin. Nutr.* **19**(1), 15–22.

McNamara, E.P., Flood, I. & Kennedy, N.P. (2001). Home tube feeding: an integrated multidisciplinary approach. *J. Hum. Nutr. Dietet.* **14**(1), 13–19.

McWhirter, J.P. & Pennington, C.R. (1994). Incidence and recognition of malnutrition in hospital. *Br. Med. J.* **308**, 945–948.

Mahony, E.H. (1973). Nutritional care of the stroke patient. *Arch. Phys. Med. Rehabil.* **54**, 569–570.

Malinow, M.R., Nieto, F.J., Kruger, W.D., Duell, P.B., Hess, D.L., Gluckman, R.A., Block, P.C., Holzgang, C.R., Anderson, P.H., Seltzer, D. et al. (1997). The effects of folic acid supplementation on plasma total homocysteine are modulated by multivitamin use and methylenetetrahydrofolate reductase genotypes. *Arterioscler. Thromb. Vasc. Biol.* **17**, 1157–1162.

Malinow, M.R., Duell, P.B., Hess, D.L., Anderson, P.H., Kruger, W.D., Phillipson, B.E., Gluckman, R.A., Block, P.C. & Upson, B.M. (1998). Reduction of plasma homocysteine levels by breakfast cereal fortified with folic acid in patients with coronary heart disease. *New Engl. J. Med.* **338**, 1009–1015.

Malinow, M.R., Bostom, A.G. & Krauss, R.M. (1999). Homocysteine, diet, and cardiovascular disease: for healthcare professionals from the Nutrition Committee, American Heart Association. *Circulation* **99**, 178–182.

Manson, J.E., Rimm, E.B., Stampfer, M.J., Colditz, G.A., Willett, W.C., Krolewski, A.S., Rosner, B., Hennekens, C.H. & Speizer, F.E. (1991). Physical activity and incidence of non-insulin-dependent diabetes mellitus in women. *Lancet* **338**, 774–778.

Manson, J.E, Stampfer, M.J., Willett, W.C., Colditz, G.A., Speizer, F.E. & Hennekens, C.H. (1993). Antioxidant vitamin consumption and incidence of stroke in women. *Circulation* **87**(2), 70 (abstract).

Manson, J.E., Willett, W.C., Stampfer, M.J., Colditz, G.A., Hunter, D.J. & Hankinson, S.E. (1995). Body weight and mortality among women. *New Engl. J. Med.* **333**, 677–685.

Martin, J., Meltzer, H. & Elliot, D. (1988). *OPCS Survey of Disability in Great Britain. Report I: The Prevalence of Disability Among Adults.* HMSO, London.

Martyn, C.N., Winter, P.D., Coles, S.J. & Edington, J. (1998). Effect of nutritional status on the use of health care resources by patients with chronic diseases living in the community. *J. Clin. Nutr.* **17**, 119–123.

Martz, D,. Rayos, G., Schielke, G.P. & Betz, A.L. (1989). Allopurinol and dimethylthiourea reduce brain infarction following middle cerebral artery occlusion in rats. *Stroke* **20**(4), 488–494.

Marx, J.J.M. (1979). Normal iron absorption and decreased red-cell iron uptake in the aged. *Blood* **53**, 204–211.

Matsumiya, N., Koehler, R.C., Kirsch, J.R. & Traystman, R.J. (1991). Conjugated superoxide dismutase reduces extent of caudate injury after transient focal ischaemia in cats. *Stroke* **22**, 1193–1200.

Matthias, D., Becker, C.H., Riezler, R. & Kindling, P.H. (1996). Homocysteine induced arteriosclerosis-like alterations of the aorta in normotensive and hypertensive rats following application of high doses of methionine. *Atherosclerosis* **122**, 201–216.

Memezawa, H., Smith, M.L. & Siesjo, B.K. (1992). Penumbral tissues salvaged by reperfusion following middle cerebral artery occlusion in rats. *Stroke* **23**, 552–559.

Metz, J., Bell, A.H., Flicker, L., Bottiglieri, T., Ibrahim, J, Seal, E., Schultz, D., Savoia, H. & McGrath, K.M. (1996). The significance of subnormal serum vitamin B12 concentration in older people. *J. Am. Geriatr. Soc.* **44**, 1355–1361.

Meydani, M. (2000). Omega-3 fatty acids alter soluble markers of endothelial function in coronary heart disease patients. *Nutr. Rev.* **58**, 56–59.

Meydani, S.N., Meydani, M., Blumberg, J.B., Leka, L.S., Siber, G., Loszewski, R., Thompson, C., Pedrosa, M.C., Diamond, R.D. & Stollar, B.D. (1997). Vitamin E supplementation and in vivo immune response in healthy elderly subjects. A randomised controlled trial. *J. Am. Med. Assoc.* **277**, 1380–1386.

Miall, W.E., Ashcroft, M.T., Lovell, H.G. & Moore, F. (1967). A longitudinal study of the decline of adult height with age in two Welsh communities. *Hum. Biol.* **39**, 445–454.

Ministry of Agriculture, Fisheries and Food (1995). *Manual of Nutrition.* 10th edn, Reference Book 342. HMSO, London.

Mirro, R., Armstaed, W.M., Mirro, J.J., Busija, D.W. & Leffler, C.W. (1989). Blood-induced superoxide anion generation on cerebral cortex of new-born pigs. *Am. J. Physiol.* **257**(26), H1560–H1564.

Mitchell, C.O.& Lipschitz, D.A. (1980). A nutritional evaluation of healthy elderly. *J. Parent. Ent. Nutr.* **4**, 603 (abstract).

Mitchell, C.O. & Lipschitz, D.A. (1982a). The effect of age and sex on routinely used measurements to assess the nutritional status of hospitalised patients. *Am. J. Clin. Nutr.* **36**, 340–349.

Mitchell, C.O. & Lipschitz, D.A. (1982b). Detection of protein–calorie malnutrition in the elderly. *Am. J. Clin. Nutr.* **35**, 398–406.

Molloy, A.M., Daly, S., Mills, J.L., Kirke, P.N., Whitehead, A.S., Ramsbottom, D., Conley, M.R., Weir, D.G. & Scot, J.M. (1997). Thermolabile variant of 5,10 methylenetetrahydrofolate reductase associated with low red-cell folates: implication for folate intake recommendations. *Lancet* **349**, 1591–1593.

Moncada, S. & Higgs, A. (1993). The L-arginine–nitric oxide pathway. *New Engl. J. Med.* **329**, 2002–2012.

Moorhouse, P.C., Grootveld, M., Halliwell, B., Quinlan, J.G. & Gutteridge, J.M.C. (1987). Allopurinol and oxypurinol are hydroxyl radical scavengers. *FEBS Lett.* **213**(1); 23–28.

Morgan, A.F., Gillum, H.L. & William, R.I. (1955). Nutritional status of the ageing. *J. Nutr.* **55**, 431–448.

Morisaki, N., Saito, I., Tamura, K., Tashiro, J., Masuda, M., Kanzaki, T., Watanabe, S., Masuda, Y. & Saito, Y. (1997). New indices of ischemic heart disease and aging: studies on the serum levels of soluble intercellular adhesion molecule-1(ICAM-1) and soluble vascular adhesion molecule-1 (VCAM-1) in patients with hypercholesterolemia and ischemic heart disease. *Atherosclerosis* **131**, 43–48.

Morley, J.E. (1986). Nutritional status of the elderly. *Am. J. Med.* **81**, 679–695.

Morley, J.E. (1993). Why do physicians fail to recognise and treat malnutrition in older persons? *J. Am. Geriatr. Soc.* **39**, 1139-1140.

Morley, J.E. (1994). Nutritional assessment is a key component of geriatric assessment. In: *Nutrition in the Elderly*, (Vellas, B.J., Guizog, Y., Garry, P.J. & Albarede, J.L. eds) Suppl. (2), pp. 5-9. Serdi, Paris.

Motoyama, T., Kawano, H., Kugiyama, K., Hirashima, O., Ohgushi, M., Tsunoda, R., Moriyama, Y., Miyao, Y., Yoshimura, M., Ogawa, H. & Yasue, H. (1998). Vitamin E administration improves impairment of endothelium-dependent vasodilation in patients with coronary spastic angina. *J. Am. Coll. Cardiol.* **32**, 1672-1679.

Mudd, S.H., Skovby, F., Levy, H.L. Pettigrew, K.D., Wilcken, B., Pyerity, R.E., Andria, G., Boers, G.H.J., Bromberg, I.L., Cerone, R. et al. (1985). The natural history of homocystinuria due to cystathionine beta-synthase deficiency. *Am. J. Hum. Genet.* **37**, 1-31.

Muhlethaler, R., Stuck, A.E., Minder, C.E., Frey, B.M. (1995). The prognostic significance of protein–energy malnutrition in geriatric patients. *Age Ageing* **24**, 193-197.

Mullen, M.J., Wright, D., Donald, A.E., Thorne, S., Thomson, H. & Deanfield, J.E. (2000). Atorvastatin but not L-arginine improves endothelial function in type I diabetes mellitus: a double-blind study. *J. Am. Coll. Cardiol.* **36**, 410-416.

Munro, H.N. & Young, V.R. (1980). Protein metabolism and requirements. In: *Metabolic and Nutritional Disorders in the Elderly*, pp. 13–25. John Wright & Sons, Bristol.

Munro, H.N., Suter, N.M. & Russell, R.M. (1987). Nutritional requirement of the elderly. *Annu. Rev. Nutr.* **7**, 23–49.

Nagel, E., Vilsendorf, A.M.Z., Bartels, M., Pichlmayr, R. (1997). Antioxidative vitamins in prevention of ischemia–reperfusion injury. *Int. J. Vit. Nutr. Res.* **67**, 298–306.

Nakayama, H., Jorgensen, H.S., Pedersen, P.M., Raaschou, H.O. & Olsen, T.S. (1997). Prevalence and risk factors for incontinence after stroke: The Copenhagen Stroke Study. *Stroke* **28**, 58–62.

National Research Council (1989). *Recommended Dietary Allowances*. 10th edn. National Academy Press, Washington DC.

Naurath, H.J., Joosten, E., Reizler, R., Stabler, S.P., Allen, R.H. & Lindenbaum, J. (1995). Effects of vitamin B12, folate and vitamin B6 supplements in elderly people with normal serum vitamin concentrations. *Lancet* **346**, 85–89.

Neaton, J.D., Blackburn, H., Jacobs, G., Kuller, L., Lee, D.J., Sherwin, R., Shih, J., Stamler, J. & Wentworth, D. (1992). Serum cholesterol level and mortality findings. *Arch. Int. Med.* **152**, 1490–1500.

Neunteufl, T., Priglinger, U., Heher, S., Zehetgrubes, M., Soregi, G., Lehr, S., Huber, K., Maurer, G., Weidinger, F. & Kostner, K. (2000). Effects of vitamin E on chronic and acute endothelial dysfunction in smokers. *J. Am. Coll. Cardiol.* **35**, 277–283.

Niittynen, L., Nurminen, M.L., Korpela, R. & Vapaatalo, H. (1999). Role of arginine, taurine and homocysteine in cardiovascular diseases. *Ann. Med.* **31**, 318–326.

Norton, B., Homer-Ward, M., Donnelly, D.M., Long, R.G. & Holmes, G.K. (1996). A randomised prospective comparison of percutaneous endoscopic gastrotomy and nasogastric tube feeding after acute dysphasic stroke. *Br. Med. J.* **312**, 13–16.

Nygard, O., Nordrehaug, J.E., Refsum, H., Ueland, P.M., Farstard, M. & Vollset, S.E. (1997). Plasma homocysteine levels and mortality in patients with coronary artery disease. *New Engl. J. Med.* **337**, 230–236.

Nyswonger, G.D. & Helmchen, R.H. (1992). Early enteral nutrition and length of stay in stroke patients. *J. Neurosci. Nurs.* **24**(4), 220–223.

Nyyssonen, K., Parvianen, M.T., Salonen, R., Tuomilehto, J. & Salonen, J.T. (1997). Vitamin C defiency and risk of myocardial infarction: prospective study of men from eastern Finland. *Br. Med. J.* **314**, 634–638.

Office of Population, Censuses and Surveys (1989). *General Household Survey 1986.* HMSO, London.

Okada, Y., Copeland, B.R., Mori, E., Tung, M.M., Thomas, W.S. & del Zoppo, G.J. (1994). P-selectin and intercellular adhesion molecule-1 expression after focal brain ischaemia and reperfusion. *Stroke* **25**, 202–211.

Omen, C.M., van Erk, M.J., Feskens, E.J., Kok, F.J. & Kromhout, D. (2000). Arginine intake and risk of coronary heart disease mortality in elderly men. *Arterioscler. Thromb. Vasc. Biol.* **20**, 2134–2139.

Omenn, G.S., Goodman, G.E., Thorquist, M.D., Balmes, J., Cullen, M.R., Glass, A., Keogh, J.P., Meyskens, F.L., Valanis, B., Williams, J.H., Barnhart, S. & Hammar, S. (1996). Effects of a combination of β carotene and vitamin A on lung cancer and cardiovascular disease. *New Engl. J. Med.* **334**, 1150–1155.

Orencia, A.J., Daviglus, M.L., Dyer, A.R., Shekelle, R.B. & Stamler, J. (1996). Fish consumption and stroke in men. *Stroke* **27**, 204–209.

Packer, L., Tritschler, H.J. & Wessel, K. (1997). Neuroprotection by the metabolic antioxidant α-lipoic acid. *Free Radix Biol. Med.* **22**, 359–378.

Patt, A., Harken, A.H., Burton, L.K., Rodell, T.C., Piermattei, D., Schorr, W.J., Parker, N.B., Berger, E.M., Horesh, I.R., Terada, L.S. et al. (1988). Xanthine oxidase-derived hydrogen peroxide contributes to ischaemia perfusion-induced oedema in gerbil brain. *J. Clin. Invest.* **81**, 1556–1562.

Pearson, T.A., LaCava, J. & Weil, H.F. (1997). Epidemiology of thrombotic-hemostatic factors and their associations with cardiovascular disease. *Am. J. Clin. Nutr.* **65**(Suppl), 1674S–1682S.

Pellegrini, N., Pareti, F.I., Stabile, F., Brusamolino, A. & Simonetti, P. (1996). Effects of moderate consumption of red wine on platelet aggregation and haemostatic variables in healthy volunteers. *Eur. J. Clin. Nutr.* **50**, 209–213.

Pellmar, T.C. & Neel, K.L. (1989). Oxidative damage in the guinea pig hippocampal slice. *Free Radical Biol. Med.* **6**, 467–472.

Perry, I.J., Refsum, H., Morris, R.W., Ebrahim, S.B., Ueland, P.M. & Shaper, A.G. (1995). Prospective study of serum total homocysteine and risk of stroke in middle aged British men. *Lancet* **346**, 1395–1398.

Peter, K., Nawroth, P., Conradt, C., Nordt, T., Weiss, T., Boehme, M., Wunsch, A., Allenberg, J., Kubler, W. & Bode, C. (1997). Circulating vascular cell adhesion molecule-l correlates with the extent of human atherosclerosis in contrast to circulating intercellular adhesion molecule-l, E-selectin, P-selectin, and thrombomodulin. *Arterioscler. Thromb. Vasc. Biol.* **17**, 505–512.

Petkau, A., Chelack, W.S., Kelly, K., Barefood, C. & Monasterski, L. (1976). Tissue distribution of bovine ^{125}I-superoxide dismutase in mice. *Res. Commun. Chem. Pathol. Pharmacol.* **15**, 641–654.

Peto, R., Doll, R., Buckley, J.D. & Sporn, M.B. (1981). Can dietary β-carotene materially reduce human cancer rates? *Nature* **290**, 201–208.

Petri, M., Roubenoff, R., Dallal, G.E. Nadeau, M.R., Selhub, J., Rosenberg, I.H. (1996). Plasma homocysteine as a risk factor for atherothrombotic events in systemic lupus erythematosus. *Lancet* **348**, 1120–1124.

Phelan, A.M. & Lange, D.G. (1990) Enhanced transport of superoxide dismutase across the blood–brain barrier using liposome encapsulated superoxide dismutase and its effect on ischaemia and reperfusion induced membrane damage. *Fed. Am. Soc. Exp. Biol. J* **4**, A896 (abstract).

Phillips, A., Shaper, A.G. & Whincup, P.H. (1989). Association between serum albumin and mortality from cardiovascular disease, cancer and other causes. *Lancet* **2**, 1434–1436.

Pitchumoni, S.S. & Doraiswamy, P.M. (1998). Current status of antioxidant therapy for Alzheimer's disease. *J. Am. Geriatr. Soc.* **46**, 1566–1572.

Poehlman, E.T. (1993). Regulation of energy expenditure in ageing humans. *J. Am. Geriatr. Soc.* **41**, 552–559.

Polidori, M.C., Frei, B., Cherubini, A., Nelles, G., Rordorf, G., Keaney, J.F. Jr, Schwamm, L., Mecocci, P., Koroshetz, W.J. & Beal, M.F. (1998). Increased plasma levels of lipid hydroperoxides in patients with ischaemic stroke. *Free Radic. Biol. Med.* **25**(4–5), 561–567.

Potter, J., Klipstein, K., Reilly, J.J. & Roberts, M. (1995). The nutritional status and clinical course of acute admissions to a geriatric unit. *Age Ageing* **24**, 131–136.

Poungvarin, N. (1998). Stroke in the developing world. *Lancet* **352**, 19–21.

Prince, R.L., Smith, M., Dick, I.M., Price, R.I., Webb, P.G., Henderson, N.K. & Harris, M.M. (1991). Prevention of postmenopausal osteoporosis: a comparative study of exercise, calcium supplementation and hormone replacement therapy. *New Engl. J. Med.* **325**(7), 1189–1195.

Pruefer, D., Scalia, R. & Lefer, A.M. (1999). Homocysteine provokes leukocyte–endothelium interaction by downregulation of nitric oxide. *Gen. Pharmacol.* **33**, 487–498.

Pryor, W.A. (2000). Vitamin E and heart disease: basic science to clinical intervention trials. *Free Radic. Biol. Med.* **28**, 141–164.

Pulsinelli, W. (1992). Pathophysiology of acute ischaemic stroke. *Lancet* **339**, 533–536.

Qureshi, A.I., Giles, W.H. & Croft, J.B. (1999). Racial differences in the incidence of intracerebral haemorrhage: effect of blood pressure and education. *Neurology* **52**, 1617–1621.

Rabeneck, L., McCullough, L.B. & Wray, N.P. (1997). Ethically justified, clinically comprehensive guidelines for percutaneous endoscopic gastrostomy tube placement. *Lancet* **349**, 496–498.

Raitakari, O.T., Adams, M.R., McCredie, R.J., Griffiths, K.A., Stocker, R. & Celermajer, D.S. (2000). Oral vitamin C and endothelial function in smokers: short-term improvement, but no sustained beneficial effect. *J. Am. Coll. Cardiol.* **35**, 1616–1621.

Rangemark, C., Hedner, J.A., Carlson, J.T., Gleerup, G. & Winther, K. (1995). Platelet function and fibrinolytic activity in hypertensive and normotensive sleep apnea patients. *Sleep* **18**, 188–194.

RANTTAS Investigators (1996). A randomised trial of tirilazad mesylate in patients with acute stroke. *Stroke* **27**, 1453–1458.

Reeds, P.J. & James, W.P.T. (1983). Protein turnover. *Lancet* **1**, 571–574.

Reinhardt, G.F., Myscofski, J.W., Wilkens, D.B., Dobin, P.G., Dobrin, P.B., Mangan, J.E.

& Stannard, R.T. (1980). Incidence and mortality of hypoalbuminemic patients in hospitalised veterans. *J. Parent. Ent. Nutr.* **4**, 357–359.

Reinhardt, R.A. (1988). Magnesium metabolism. *Arch. Int. Med.* **148**, 2415–2420.

Rennie, M. & Harrison, R. (1984). Effect of injury, disease and malnutrition on protein metabolism in man. Unanswered questions. *Lancet* **1**, 323–325.

Rich, M.W., Keller, A.J., Schechtman, K.B., Marshall, W.G. Jr & Kouchoukos, N.T. (1989). Increased complications and prolonged hospital stay in elderly cardiac surgical patients with low serum albumin. *Am. J. Cardiol.* **63**, 714–718.

Ridker, P.M., Hennekens, C.H., Roitman-Johnson, B., Stampfer, M.J. & Allen, J. (1998). Plasma concentration of soluble intercellular adhesion molecule 1 and risks of future myocardial infarction in apparently healthy men. *Lancet* **351**, 88–92.

Riemersma, R.A., Wood, D.A. Macintyre, C.C.A., Elton, R.A., Gey, K.F. & Oliver, M.F. (1991). Risk of angina pectoris and plasma concentrations of vitamin A, C, E and carotene. *Lancet* **337**, 1–5.

Rimm, E.B., Stampfer, M.J., Ascherio, A., Giovannucci, E., Colditz, G.A. & Willett, W.C. (1993). Vitamin E consumption and the risk of coronary heart disease in men. *New Engl. J. Med.* **328**, 1450–1460.

Rimm, E.B., Willett, W.C. Hu, F.B., Sampson, L., Colditz, G.A., Manson, J.E., Hennekens, C. & Stampfer, M.J. (1998). Folate and vitamin B6 from diet and supplements in relation to risk of coronary heart disease among women. *J. Am. Med. Assoc.* **279**, 359–364.

Roberts, S.H., James, O. & Jarvis, E.H. (1977). Bacterial overgrowth syndrome without 'blind loop', a cause for malnutrition in the elderly. *Lancet* **ii**, 1193–1195.

Robinson, K., Arheart, K., Refsum, H., Brattstrom, L., Boers, G., Ueland, P., Rubba, P., Palma-Reis, R., Meleady, R., Daly, L., Witteman, J. & Graham, I. (1998). Low circulating folate and vitamin B6 concentrations: risk factors for stroke, peripheral vascular disease, and coronary artery disease: European COMAC Group. *Circulation* **97**, 437–443.

Rolland-Cachera, M.F., Cole, T.J., Sempe, M., Tichet, J., Rossignol, C. & Charraud, A. (1991). Body mass index variations: centiles from birth to 87 years. *Eur. J. Clin. Nutr.* **45**, 13–21.

Ross, R. (1999). Atherosclerosis: an inflammatory disease. *New Eng. J. Med.* **340**, 115–149.

Rothschild, M.A., Horatz, M. & Schriber, S.S. (1972a). Albumin synthesis (first of two parts). *New Engl. J. Med.* **286**, 748–757.

Rothschild, M.A., Horatz, M. & Schriber, S.S. (1972b). Albumin synthesis (second of two parts). *New Engl. J. Med.* **286**, 816–820.

Rothwell, N.J., Stock, M.J. (1983). Effect of age on diet-induced thermogenesis and brown adipose tissue metabolism in the rat. *Int. J. Obesity* **7**, 583–589.

Royal College of Physicians (1991). *Medical Aspects of Exercise: Benefits and Risks.* Royal College of Physicians, London.

Rudman, D., Feller, A.G., Nagraj, H.S., Jackson, D.L., Rudman, I.W. & Mattson, D.E. (1987). Relation of serum albumin concentration to death rate in nursing home men. *J. Parent. Ent. Nutr.* **11**, 360–363.

Russell, R.M. (1986). Implications of gastric atrophy for vitamin and mineral nutriture. In: *Nutrition and Ageing* (Hutchinson, M.L. & Munro, H.N. eds), p. 59. Harcourt Brace Jovanovich, San Diego.

Russell, R.M. (1988). Malabsorption and ageing. In: *Ageing in Liver and Gastrointestinal Tract* (Bianchi, L., Holt, P., James, O.F.W. & Butler, R.N., eds), 47 Falk Symposium. pp. 297–307. Kluwer Academic, Lancaster.

Russell, R.M. & Suter, P.M. (1993). Vitamin requirements of elderly people: an update. *Am. J. Clin. Nutr.* **58**, 4–14.

Ryan, M., Grayson, L. & Clarke, D.J. (1997). The total antioxidant capacity of human serum measured using enhanced chemiluminescence is almost completely accounted for by urate. *Ann. Clin. Biochem.* **34**, 688–689.

Salem, M., Kasinski, N., Andrei, A.M., Brussel, T., Gold, M.R., Conn, A. & Chernow, B. (1991). Hypomagnesemia is a frequent finding in the emergency department in patients with chest pains. *Arch. Int. Med.* **151**, 2185–2190.

Sandstrom, B., Alhaug, J., Einarsdottir, K., Simpura, E.M. & Isaksson, B. (1985). Nutritional status, energy and protein intake in general medical patients in three Nordic hospitals. *Hum. Nutr. Appl. Nutr.* **39A**, 87–94.

Sano, M., Ernesto, C., Thomas, R.G., Klauber, M.R., Schafer, K., Grundman, M., et al. (1997). A controlled trial of selegiline, alpha-tocopherol, or both as a treatment for Alzheimer's disease. *New Engl. J. Med.* **336**, 1216–1222.

Savage, D.G., Lindenbaum, J., Stabler, S.P. & Allen, R.H. (1994). Sensitivity of serum methylmalonic acid and total homocysteine determinants for diagnosing cobalamin and folate deficiencies. *Am. J. Med.* **96**, 239–246.

Schiffman, S.S. (1973). In: *Mental Illness in Later Life* (Busse, E.W. & Pfeiffer, E. eds), p. 269. American Psychiatric Association, Washington DC.

Schiffman, S.S. (1978). Changes in taste and smell in old persons. In: *Advances in Research*, Vol. 2, pp. 1–6. Duke University Center for the Study of Ageing and Human Development, Durham, N.C.

Schmidley, J.W. (1990). Free radicals in central nervous system ischaemia. *Stroke* **21**, 1086–1090.

Schmidt, H.H., Nau, H., Wittfoht, W., Gerlach, J., Prescher, K.E., Klein, M.M., Niroomand, F. & Bohme, E. (1988). Arginine is a physiological precursor of endothelium-derived nitric oxide. *Eur. J. Pharmacol.* **154**, 213–216.

Schofield, W.N., Schofield, C. & James, W.P.T. (1985). Basal metabolic rate – review and prediction. *Hum. Nutr. Clin. Nutr.* **39C**(Suppl), 1–96.

Schorah, C.J., Tormey, W.P., Brooks, G.H., Robertshaw, A.M., Young, A.M., Talukder, R. & Kelly, J.F. (1981). The effect of vitamin C supplements on body weight, serum protein, and general health of an elderly population. *Am. J. Clin. Nutr.* **34**, 871–876.

Selhub, J., Jacques, P.F., Wilson, P.W., Rush, D. & Rosenberg, I.H. (1993). Vitamin status and intake as primary determinants of homocysteinemia in an elderly population. *J. Am. Med. Assoc.* **270**, 2693–2698.

Seljeflot, I., Arnesen, H., Brude, I.R., Nenseter, M.S., Drevon, C.A. & Hjermann, I. (1998). Effects of omega-3 fatty acids and/or antioxidants on endothelial cell markers. *Eur. J. Clin. Invest.* **28**, 629–635.

Seltzer, M.H., Bashidas, J.A. & Cooper, D.M. (1979). Instant nutritional assessment. *J. Parent. Ent. Nutr.* **3**, 157–159.

Senapati, A., Jenner, G., Thompson, R.P.H. (1989). Zinc in the elderly. *Q. J. Med.* **70**, 81–87.

Shenkin, A. & Steele, W. (1978). Clinical and laboratory assessment of protein status. *Proc. Nutr. Soc.* **37**, 95–103.

Shike, M., Russel, D.M., Detsky, A.S., Harrison, J.E., McNeill, K.G., Shepherd, F.A., Feld, R., Evans, W.K. & Jeejeebhoy, K.N. (1984). Changes in body composition in patients with small-cell lung cancer. The effect of total parenteral nutrition as an adjunct to chemotherapy. *Ann. Int. Med.* **101**(3), 303–309.

Shimokawa, H. (1999). Primary endothelial dysfunction: atherosclerosis. *J. Mol. Cell. Cardiol.* **31**, 23–27.

Shiu, G.K. & Nemoto, E.M. (1981). Barbiturate attenuation of brain fatty acid liberation during global ischaemia. *J. Neurosurg.* **37**, 1448–1456.

Siesjo, B.K. (1984). Cerebral circulation and metabolism. *J. Neurosurg.* **60**, 883–908.

Siesjo, B.K. (1992a). Pathophysiology and treatment of focal cerebral ischaemia, part 1. *J. Neurosurg.* **77**, 169–184.

Siesjo, B.K. (1992b). Pathophysiology and treatment of focal cerebral ischaemia, part 2. Mechanisms of damage and treatment. *J. Neurosurg.* **77**, 337–354.

Simons, L.A., von Konigsmark, M., Simons, J., Stocker, R. & Celermajer, D.S. (1999). Vitamin E ingestion does not improve arterial endothelial dysfunction in older adults. *Atherosclerosis* **143**, 193–199.

Sjogren, A., Osterberg, T. & Steen, B. (1994). Intake of energy, nutrients and food: a population study of Swedish people. *Age Ageing* **23**, 108–112.

Skyrme-Jones, R.A., O'Brien, R.C., Berry, K.L. & Meredith, I.T. (2000). Vitamin E supplementation improves endothelial function in type I diabetes mellitus: a randomized, placebo-controlled study. *J. Am. Coll. Cardiol.* **36**, 94–102.

Souba, W.W. (1997). Nutritional support. *New Engl. J. Med.* **336**, 41–47.

Southgate, D.A.T. & Durnin, J.V.G.A. (1970). Carlorie conversion factors. An experimental reassessment of the factors used in the calculation of the energy value of human diets. *Br. J. Nutr.* **24**, 517–535.

Spitzer, M.E. (1988). Taste acuity in institutionalised and non-institutionalised elderly men. *J. Gerontol.* **43**, 71–74.

Springer, T.A. (1994). Traffic signals for lymphocyte recirculation and leukocyte emigration: the multistep paradigm. *Cell* **76**, 301–314.

Stableforth, P.G. (1986). Supplement feeds and nitrogen and calorie balance following femoral neck fracture. *Br. J. Surg.* **73**, 651–655.

Stampfer, M.J., Malinow, R., Willett, W.C., Newcomer, L.M., Upson, B., Ullman, D., Tishler, P.V. & Hennekens, C.H. (1992). A prospective study of plasma homocysteine and risk of myocardial infarction in US physicians. *J. Am. Med. Assoc.* **268**, 877–881.

Stampfer, M.J., Hennekens, C.H., Manson, J.E., Colditz, G.A., Rosner, B. & Willett, W.C. (1993). Vitamin E consumption and the risk of coronary disease in women. *New Eng. J. Med.* **328**, 1444–1449.

Steinberg, D. (2000). Is there a potential therapeutic role for vitamin E or other antioxidants in atherosclerosis? *Curr. Opin. Lipidol.* **11**(6), 603–607.

Stephens, N.G., Parsons, A., Schofield, P.M., Kelly, F., Cheeseman, K. & Mitchinson, M.J. (1996). Randomized controlled trial of vitamin E in patients with coronary disease: Cambridge Heart Antioxidant Study (CHAOS). *Lancet* **347**, 781–786.

Stewart-Lee, A.L., Forster, L.A., Nourooz-Zadeh, J., Ferns, G.A. & Anggard, E.E. (1994).

Vitamin E protects against impairment of endothelium-mediated relaxations in cholesterol-fed rabbits. *Arterioscler. Thromb.* **14**, 494–499.

Still, R.A. & McDowell, I.F. (1998). Clinical implications of plasma homocysteine measurement in cardiovascular disease. *J. Clin. Pathol.* **51**, 183–188.

Stroes, E.S., van Faasen, E.E., Yo, M., Martasek, P., Boer, P., Govers, R. & Rabelink, T.J. (2000). Folic acid reverts dysfunction of endothelial nitric oxide synthase. *Circ. Res.* **86**, 1129–1134.

Suarna, C., Dean, R.T., May, J. & Stocker, R. (1995). Human atherosclerosic plaque contains both oxidized lipids and relatively large amounts of alpha-tocopherol and ascorbate. *Arterioscler. Throm. Vasc. Biol.* **15**, 1616–1624.

Sullivan, D.H. & Walls, R.C. (1994). Impact of nutritional status on morbidity in a population of geriatric rehabilitation patients. *J. Am. Geriatr. Soc.* **42**, 471–477.

Sullivan, D.H., Walls, R.C. & Bopp, M.M. (1995). Protein–energy undernutrition and the risk of mortality. *J. Am. Geriatr. Soc.* **43**, 507–512.

Sun, G.U., Tang, W., Huang, S.F. & Foudin, L. (1984). Is phosphatidylinositol involved in the release of fatty acids in cerebral ischaemia? In: *Inositol and Phosphoinositides: Metabolism and Biological Regulation* (Bleasdale, J.E., Eichberg, J. & Hauser-Clifton, N.J., eds), pp. 511–527. Humana Press, Totowa, NJ.

Suter, P.M. (1999). The effects of potassium, magnesium, calcium and fiber on risk of stroke. *Nutr. Rev.* **57**, 84–88.

Syme, S.I., Marmot, M.G., Kagan, A., Rato, H. & Rhoads, G. (1975). Epidemiological studies of coronary heart disease and stroke. *Am. J. Epidemiol.* **102**, 477–480.

Tawakol, A., Omland, T., Gerhard, M., Wu, J.T. & Creager, M.A. (1997). Hyperhomocyst(e)inemia is associated with impaired endothelium-dependent vasodilation in humans. *Circulation* **95**, 1119–1121.

Tayback, M., Kumanyika, S. & Chee, E. (1990). Body weight as a risk factor in the elderly. *Arch. Int. Med.* **150**, 1065–1072.

Taylor, G.G. (1980). A clinical survey of elderly people from a nutritional standpoint. In: *Vitamins in the Elderly* (Exton-Smith, A.N. & Scott, D.L., eds), pp. 51–56. John Wright, Bristol.

Theilmeier, G., Chan, J.R., Zalpour, C., Anderson, B., Wang, B.Y., Wolf, A., Tsao, P.S. & Cooke, J.P. (1997). Adhesiveness of mononuclear cells in hypercholesterolemic humans is normalized by dietary L-arginine. *Arterioscler. Thromb. Vasc. Biol.* **17**, 3557–3564.

Thomas, A.J., Bunker, V.W., Hinks, L.J., Sodha, M., Mullee, M.A. & Clayton, B.E. (1988). Energy, protein, zinc and copper status of twenty one elderly inpatients: analysed dietary intake and biochemical indices. *Br. J. Clin. Nutr.* **59**, 181–191.

Thomas, A.J., Bunker, V.W., Stansfield, M.F., Sodha, N.K. & Clayton, B.E. (1989). Iron status of hospitalised and house bound elderly people. *Q. J. Med.* **70**, 175–184.

Thornton, J., Symes, C. & Heaton, K. (1983). Moderate alcohol intake reduces bile cholesterol saturation and raises HDL cholesterol. *Lancet* **2**, 819–822.

Ting, H.H., Timimi, F.K., Haley, E.A., Roddy, M.A., Ganz, P. & Creager, M.A. (1997). Vitamin C improves endothelium-dependent vasodilation in forearm resistance vessels of humans with hypercholesterolemia. *Circulation* **95**, 2617–2622.

Tobian, L., Lange, J., Ulm, K., Wold, L. & Iwai, J. (1985). Potassium reduces cerebral haemorrhage and death rate in hypertensive rats, even when blood pressure is not lowered. *Hypertension* **7** (Suppl 1), 1-110–1-114.

Todd, J.E. & Walker, A.M. (1980). *Adult Dental Health, Vol. 1, England and Wales, 1968–1978.* HMSO, London.

Tornwall, M.E., Virtamo, J., Haukka, J.K., et al. (1999). The effect of alpha-tocopherol and beta-carotene supplementation on symptoms and progression of intermittent claudication in a controlled trial. *Atherosclerosis* **147**, 193–197.

Tortora, G.J. & Grabowski, S.R. (1996). *Principles of Anatomy and Physiology*, 8th edn. p. 424. Harper Collins, London.

Traystamn, R.J., Kirsch, J.R. & Koehler, R.C. (1991). Oxygen radical mechanism of brain injury following ischaemia and reperfusion. *J. Appl. Physiol.* **71**(4), 1185–1195.

Treasure, J. & Ploth, D. (1983). Role of dietary potassium in the treatment of hypertension. *Hypertension* **5**, 864–872.

Truswell, A.S. (1979). Historical perspective. In: *Human Nutrition and Dietetics* (Davidson, S., Passmore, R., Brock, J.F. & Truswell, A.S., eds) pp. 1–5. Churchill Livingstone, Edinburgh.

Tsai, J.C., Perrella, M.A., Yoshizumi, M., Hsieh, C.M., Haber, E., Schlegal, R. & Lee, M.E. (1994). Promotion of vascular smooth muscle growth by homocysteine: a link to atherosclerosis. *Proc. Natl. Acad. Sci. USA* **91**, 6369–6373.

Tsao, P.S., Buitrago, R., Chan, J.R. & Cooke, J.P. (1996). Fluid flow inhibits endothelial adhesiveness: nitric oxide and transcriptional regulation of VCAM-l. *Circulation* **94**, 1682–1689.

Turrens, J.F., Crapo, J.D. & Freeman, B.A. (1984). Protection against oxygen toxicity by intravenous injection of liposome-entrapped catalase and superoxide dismutase. *J. Clin. Invest.* **73**, 87–95.

Uauy, R., Scrimshaw, N.S. & Young, V.R. (1978). Human protein requirement: nitrogen balance response to graded levels of egg protein in elderly men and women. *Am. J. Clin. Nutr.* **31**, 779–785.

Ueland P.M. (1995). Homocysteine species as components of plasma redox thiol status. *Clin. Chem.* **41**, 340–342.

Ueland, P.M., Refsum, H., Beresford, S.A.A. & Vollset, S.E. (2000). The controversy over homocysteine and cardiovascular risk. *J. Clin. Nutr.* **72**, 324–332.

Ullegaddi, R., Powers, H.J. & Gariballa, S.E. (2002). A randomised controlled trial of vitamin E and C supplementation following acute ischaemic stroke. Presentation at the European Society of Parenteral and Enteral Nutrition Meeting, Glasgow, 2002.

Unosson, M., Ek, A.C., Bjurulf, P., von Schenck, H. & Larsson, J. (1994). Feeding dependence and nutritional status after acute stroke. *Stroke* **25**, 366–371.

Usui, M., Matsuoka, H., Miyazaki, H., Ueda, S., Okuda, S. & Imaizumi, T. (1999). Endothelial dysfunction by acute hyperhomocyst(e)inaemia: restoration by folic acid. *Clin. Sci. (Colch)* **96**, 235–239.

Van den Berg, M. Boers, G.H., Franken, D.G., Blom, H.J., Van Kamp, G.J., Jakobs, C., Rauwerda, J.A., Kluft, C. & Stehouwert, C.D. (1995). Hyperhomocysteinaemia and endothelial dysfunction in young patients with peripheral arterial occlusive disease. *Eur. J. Clin. Invest.* **25**, 176–181.

Vane, J.R., Born, G.V.R. & Welzel, D. (eds) (1995). *The Endothelial Cell in Health and Disease.* Schattauer, Stuttgart.

Van Wylen, D.G., Park, T.S., Rubio, R. & Berne, R.M. (1986). Increases in interstitial fluid adenosine concentration during hypoxia, local potassium infusion and ischaemia. *J. Cereb. Blood Flow Metab.* **6**, 522–528.

Vartiainen, E., Sarti, E., Tuomilehto, J. & Kuulasmaa, K. (1995). Do changes in cardiovascular risk factors explain changes in mortality from stroke in Finland? *Br. Med. J.* **310**, 901–904.

Verges, B.L. (1999). Dyslipidemia in diabetes mellitus. *Diabet. Metab.* **25**, 32–40.

Verhaar, M.C., Wever, R.M., Kastelein, J.J., van Dam, T., Koomans, H.A. & Rabelink, T.J. (1998). 5-Methyltetrahydrofolate, the active form of folic acid, restores endothelial function in familial hypercholesterolemia. *Circulation* **97**, 237–241.

Verhaar, M.C., Wever, R.M., Kastelein, J.J., van Loon, D., Milstein, S., Koomans, H.A. & Rabelink, T.J. (1999). Effects of oral folic acid supplementation on endothelial function in familial hypercholesterolemia. A randomised placebo-controlled trial. *Circulation* **100**, 335–338.

Verhoef, P., Hennekens, C.H., Malinow, M.R., Kok, F.J., Willet, W.C. & Stampfer, M.J. (1994). A prospective study of plasma homocysteine and risk of ischaemic stroke. *Stroke* **25**, 1924–1930.

Verhoef, P., Stampfer, M.J., Buring, J.E., Gaziano, J.M., Allen, R.H., Stabler, S.P., Reynolds, R.D., Kok, F.J., Hennekens, C.H. & Willet, W.C. (1996). Homocysteine metabolism and risk of myocardial infarction: relation with vitamin B6, B12, and folate. *Am. J. Epidemiol.* **143**, 845–859.

Verhoef, P., Hennekens, C.H., Allen, R.H., Stabler, S.P., Willet, W.C. & Stampfer, M.J. (1997). Plasma total homocysteine and risk of angina pectoris with subsequent coronary artery bypass surgery. *Am. J. Cardiol.* **79**, 799–801.

Vermeulen, E.G., Stenhouwer, C.D., Twisk, J.W., van den Berg, M., de Jong, S.C., Mackaay, A.J., van Campen, C.M., Visser, F.C., Jakobs, C.A., Bulterjis, E.J. & Rauwerda, J.A. (2000a). Effect of homocysteine-lowering treatment with folic acid plus vitamin B6 on progression of subclinical atherosclerosis: a randomized, placebo-controlled trial. *Lancet* **355**, 517–522.

Vermeulen, E.G., Rauwerda, J.A., Erix, P., de Jong, S.C., Twisk, J.W., Jakobs, C., Witjes, R.J. & Stehouwer, C.D. (2000b). Normohomocysteinaemia and vitamin-treated hyperhomocysteinaemia are associated with similar risks of cardiovascular events in patients with premature atherothrombotic cerebrovascular disease. A prospective cohort study. *Neth. J. Med.* **56**, 138–146.

Verschuren, W.M.M., Jacobs, D.R., Bloemberg, B.P.M., Kromhout, D., Menotti, A., Aravanis, C., Blackburn, H., Buzina, R., Dontas, A.S. & Fidanza, F. (1995). Serum total cholesterol and long-term coronary heart disease mortality in different cultures. Twenty-five year follow up of the seven country study. *J. Am. Med. Assoc.* **274**, 131–136.

Viteri, F.E. & Alvarado, J. (1970). The creatinine height index: its use in the estimation of the degree of protein depletion and repletion in protein calorie malnourished children. *Paediatrics* **46**, 696–706.

Vogel, R.A. (1997). Coronary risk factors, endothelial function and atherosclerosis: a review. *Clin. Cardiol.* **20**, 426–432.

von Shacky, C. (2000). n-3 Fatty acids and the prevention of coronary atherosclerosis. *Am. J. Clin. Nutr.* **71**(Suppl), 224S–227S.

Wade, D.T. (1992). Stroke: rehabilitation. *Lancet* **339**, 791–793.

Wade, D.T., Hewer, R.L., Skilbeck, C.E., & David, R.M. (eds) (1985). *Stroke: A Critical Approach*. Chapman and Hall, London.

Wagner, P.A., Jernigan, J.A., Bailey, L.B., Nickens, C. & Brazzi, G.A. (1983). Zinc nutriture and cell mediated immunity in the aged. *Int. J. Vit. Nutr. Res.* **53**, 94–101.

Wald, N.J., Watt, H.C., Law, M.R., Weir, D.G., McPartlin, J. & Scott, J.M. (1998). Homocysteine and ischemic heart disease: results of a prospective study with implications regarding prevention. *Arch. Int. Med.* **158**, 862–867.

Wang, J.S., Jen, C.J. & Chen, H.I. (1995). Effects of exercise training and deconditioning on platelet function in men. *Arterioscler. Thromb. Vasc. Biol.* **15**, 1668–1674.

Waring, W.S. (2002). Uric acid: an important antioxidant in acute ischaemic stroke. *Q. J. Med.* **95**, 691–693.

Waring, W.S., Webb, D.J. & Maxwell, S.R. (2001). Systemic uric acid administration increases serum antioxidant capacity in healthy volunteers. *J. Cardiovasc. Pharmacol.* **38**, 365–371.

Warlow, C.P., Dennis, M.S., van Gijn, J., Hankey, G.J., Sandercock, P.A.G., Bamford, J.M. & Wardlaw, J. (1996). Reducing the burden of stroke and improving the public health. In: *Stroke: A Practical Guide to Management* (Warlow, C.P., Dennis, M.S., van Gijn, J., Hankey, G.J., Sandercock, P.A.G., Bamford, J.M. & Wardlaw, J. eds), pp. 395, 632–649. Blackwell Science, Oxford.

Weber, C., Erl, W., Pietsch, A., Danesch, U. & Weber, P. (1995). Docosahexaenoic acid selectively attenuates induction of vascular cell adhesion molecule-1 and subsequent monocytic adhesion to human endothelial cells stimulated by tumor necrosis factor-alpha. *Arterioscler. Thromb. Vasc. Biol.* **15**, 622–628.

Weber, C., Erl, W., Weber, K. & Weber, P.C. (1996). Increased adhesiveness of isolated monocytes to endothelium is prevented by vitamin C intake in smokers. *Circulation* **93**, 1488–1492.

Wei, E.P., Christman, C.W., Kontos, H.A. & Povlishock, J.T. (1985). Effects of oxygen radicals on cerebral arterioles. *Am. J. Physiol.* **248**(17), H157–H162.

Weinsier, R.L. & Heimburger, D.C. (1997). Distinguishing malnutrition from disease: the search goes on. *Am. J. Clin. Nutr.* **66**, 1063–1064.

Welch, G.N., Upchurch, G. Jr & Loscalzo, J. (1997). Hyperhomocyst(e)inaemia and atherothrombosis. *Ann. N. Y. Acad. Sci.* **811**, 48–58.

Westerberg, E., Deshpande, J.K. & Wieloch, T. (1987). Regional differences in arachidonic acid release in rat hippocampal CA1 and CA3 regions during cerebral ischaemia. *J. Cereb. Blood Flow Metab.* **7**, 189–192.

Westergren, A., Karlsson, S., Andersson, P., Ohlsson, O. & Hallberg, I.R. (2001). Eating difficulties, need for assisted eating, nutritional status and pressure ulcers in patients admitted for stroke rehabilitation. *J. Clin. Nurs.* **10**(2), 257–269.

White, B.C., Hildebrandt, J.F., Evans, A.T., Aronson, L., Indrieri, R.J., Hoehner, T., Fox, L., Huang, R. & Johns, D. (1985). Prolonged cardiac arrest and resuscitation in dogs: brain mitochondrial function with different artificial perfusion methods. *Ann. Emerg. Med.* **14**, 383–388.

Wieloch, T. & Siesjo, B.K. (1982). Ischaemic brain injury: the importance of calcium, lipolytic activities, and fatty acids. *Path. Biol.* **30**, 269–277.

Williams, C.M., Driver, L.T., Older, J. & Dickerson, J.W. (1989). A controlled trial of sip-feed supplements in elderly orthopaedic patients. *Eur. J. Clin. Nutr.* **43**, 267–274.

Williams, P.T. (1996). High-density lipoprotein cholesterol and other risk factors for coronary heart disease in female runners. *New Engl. J. Med.* **334**, 1298–1303.

Wilmink, H.W., Stroes, E.S., Erkelens, W.D., Gerritsen, W.B., Wever, R., Banga, J.D. & Rabelink, T.J. (2000). Influence of folic acid on postprandial endothelial dysfunction. *Arterioscler. Thromb. Vasc. Biol.* **20**, 185–188.

Woo, J., Ho, S.C., Mak, Y.T., Law, L.K. & Cheung, A. (1994). Nutritional status of elderly patients during recovery from chest infection and the role of nutritional supplements. *Age Ageing* **23**, 40–48.

Woo, K.S., Chook, P., Lolin, Y.I., Cheung, A.S., Chan, L.T., Sun, Y.Y., Sanderson, J.E., Metreweli, C. & Celermajer, D.S. (1997). Hyperhomocyst(e)inemia is a risk factor for arterial endothelial dysfunction in humans. *Circulation* **96**, 2542–2544.

Woo, K.S., Chook, P., Lolin, Y.I., Sanderson, J.E., Metreweli, C. & Celermajer, D.S. (1999). Folic acid improves arterial endothelial function in adults with hyperhomocystinemia. *J. Am. Coll. Cardiol.* **34**, 2002–2006.

Woodside, J.V., Yarnell, J.W.G., McMaster, D., Young, I.S., Harmon, D.L., McCrum, E.E., Patterson, C.C., Gey, K.F., Whitehead, A.S. & Evans, A. (1998). Effect of B-group vitamins and antioxidant vitamins on hyperhomocysteinaemia: a double-blind, randomised, factorial-design, controlled trial. *Am. J. Clin. Nutr.* **67**, 858–866.

World Health Organization (1971). *Cerebrovascular Disease Prevention, Treatment and Rehabilitation.* Technical Report Series No. 469. WHO, Geneva.

World Health Organization (1985). *Energy and Protein Requirements. Report of a Joint FAO/WHO/UNU Expert Consultation.* Technical Report Series No. 724. WHO, Geneva.

World Health Organization (1989). *The WHO MONICA Project.* World Health Stat Q 42, pp. 27–149.

Wu, D., Koga, T., Martin, K.R. & Meydani, M. (1999). Effect of vitamin E on human aortic endothelial cell production of chemokines and adhesion to monocytes. *Atherosclerosis* **147**, 297–307.

Xie, J.X., Sasak, S., Joossens, J.V. & Kesteloot, H. (1992). The relationship between urinary cations obtained from the INTERSALT study and cerebrovascular mortality. *J. Hum. Hypertension* **6**, 17–21.

Yamamoto, M., Shima, T., Uozumi, T., Sogabe, T., Yamada, K. & Kawasaki, T. (1983). A possible role of lipidperoxidation in cellular damages caused by cerebral ischemia and the protective effect of a-tocopherol administration. *Stroke* **14**, 977–982.

Yamori, Y. (1987). Hypertensive cerebrovascular disease: importance of nutrition in pathogenesis and prevention. *Ann. N.Y. Acad. Sci.* 92–103.

Yamori, Y., Nara, Y., Mizushima, S., Sawamura, M. & Horie, R. (1994). Nutritional factors for stroke and major cardiovascular diseases: international epidemiological comparison of dietary prevention. *Health Rep.* **6**(1), 22–27.

Yochum, L.A., Folsom, A.R. & Kushi, L.H. (2000). Intake of antioxidant vitamins and risk of death from stroke in postmenopausal women. *Am. J. Clin. Nutr.* **72**(2), 476–478.

Yoshida, S., Inoh, S., Asano, T., Sano, K., Kubota, M., Shimazaki, H. & Ueta, N. (1980). Effects of transient ischaemia on fatty acids and phospholipids in the gerbil brain. *J. Neurosurg.* **53**, 323–331.

Yoshida, S., Abe, K., Busto, R., Watson, B.D., Kogure, K. & Ginsberg, M.D. (1982). Influence of transient ischaemia on lipid-soluble antioxidants, fatty acids and energy metabolites in rat brain. *Brain Res.* **245**, 307–316.

Yoshida, B., Busto, R., Santiso, M. & Ginsberg, M.D. (1984). Brain lipid peroxidation induced by postischaemic reoxygenation in vitro: effect of vitamin E. *J. Cereb. Blood Flow Metab.* **4**, 466–469.

Young, B., Ott, L., Twyman, D., Norton, J., Rapp, R., Tibbs, P., Haack, D., Brivins, B. & Dempsey, R. (1987). The effect of nutritional support on outcome from severe head injury. *J. Neurosurg.* **67**, 668-676.

Yu, A.C.H., Chan, P.H. & Fishman, R.A. (1986). Effects of arachidonic acid on glutamate and gamma-aminobutyric acid uptake in primary cultures of rat cerebral cortical astrocytes and neurons. *J. Neurochem.* **47**, 1181–1189.

Yusuf, S., Dagenais, G., Pogue, J., Bosch, J. & Sleight, P. (2000). Vitamin E supplementation and cardiovascular events in high-risk patients. The Heart Outcomes Prevention Evaluation Study Investigators. *New Engl. J. Med.* **342**, 154–160.

Zhang, J., Sasaki, S., Amano, K. & Kesteloot, H. (1999). Fish consumption and mortality from all causes, ischaemic heart disease, and stroke: an ecological study. *Prev. Med.* **28**, 520–529.

Zhang, X.M. & Ellis, E.F. (1990). Superoxide dismutase reduces permeability and oedema induced by hypertension in rats. *Am. J. Physiol.* **259**(28), H497-H503.

Index